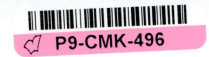
Teach Your Child
Meditation

Teach Your Child
Meditation

70 Fun & Easy Ways to Help Kids
De-Stress and Chill Out

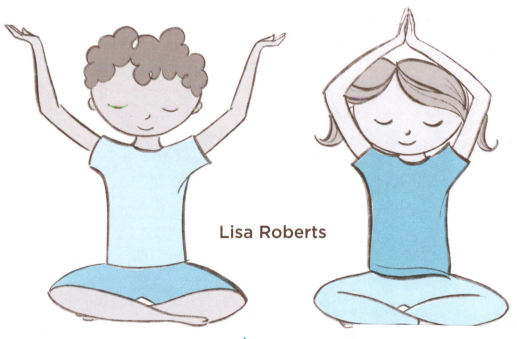

Lisa Roberts

STERLING
New York

STERLING
New York

An Imprint of Sterling Publishing Co., Inc.
1166 Avenue of the Americas
New York, NY 10036

ISBN 978-1-4549-2918-5

Library of Congress Cataloging-in-Publication Data

Names: Roberts, Lisa (Yoga instructor), author.
Title: Teach your child meditation : 70 fun & easy ways to help kids
  de-stress and chill out / Lisa Roberts.
Other titles: Breathe, chill
Description: New York : Sterling Publishing, [2018] | Includes
  bibliographical references and index.
Identifiers: LCCN 2018001262 | ISBN 9781454929185 (pbk.)
Subjects: LCSH: Breathing exercises. | Meditation for children. | Stress
  management for children. | Mind and body. | Relaxation--Technique.
Classification: LCC RA782 .R6324 2018 | DDC 613/.192--dc23
LC record available at https://lccn.loc.gov/2018001262

Distributed in Canada by Sterling Publishing Co., Inc.
^{c}/o Canadian Manda Group, 664 Annette Street
Toronto, Ontario M6S 2C8, Canada
Distributed in the United Kingdom by GMC Distribution Services
Castle Place, 166 High Street, Lewes, East Sussex BN7 1XU, England
Distributed in Australia by NewSouth Books
45 Beach Street, Coogee, NSW 2034, Australia

For information about custom editions, special sales, and premium and corporate purchases, please contact
Sterling Special Sales at 800-805-5489 or specialsales@sterlingpublishing.com.

Manufactured in Canada

2 4 6 8 10 9 7 5 3 1

sterlingpublishing.com

Cover design by Elizabeth Mihaltse Lindy
Interior design by Shannon Nicole Plunkett
Illustrations by Julia Morris

Teach Your Child Meditation is dedicated to those who dare
to teach beyond the mind and awaken the soul.

Cont

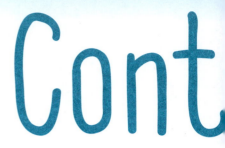

PART ONE:
I'm the Boss of My Breath

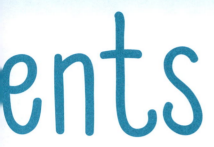

ents

Introduction

Overloaded with schoolwork, extracurricular activities, responsibilities, and expectations, today's children are busy and stressed out. Buzzing around in "go" mode is physically and mentally exhausting; it's not a healthy state for anybody, and kids especially need to rest their developing minds and bodies. Yet many children do not know how to slow things down or simply relax.

Wouldn't it be beneficial to equip our children with the skills to help them cope with stress? Imagine the value of teaching your kids how to meditate—providing them with the tools, knowledge, and ability to self-regulate, concentrate, and respond to stressful or difficult situations in a healthy and positive manner. It's not as challenging as you may think.

Teach Your Child Meditation features seventy fun and effective activities to engage kids in meditation practice. No, your child may not sit in lotus position, quietly chanting "Om" for thirty minutes—not many children would—but he or she may happily play a focus-based game with a partner for ten minutes and not think about anything else the entire time. In yoga, this is called single-pointed focus, or meditation.

I developed the creative games and activities presented in this book to appeal to kids of all ages, regardless of yoga or meditation experience. Working as a pediatric yoga specialist at a major children's hospital teaching critically ill, disabled, and hospitalized children ages two to twenty-one, I quickly learned to adapt traditional yoga and meditation techniques to make them accessible and appealing to children.

We have so much fun playing and exploring that many of my patients have no idea they are doing something good for them! It's at the end of our sessions (or during, if they blurt out "This feels great!" or "I feel so relaxed!"), when we reflect on how they feel, that they begin to realize breathing and meditation is something they can practice on their own—to aid in pain control and anxiety during their hospital stay and in their daily lives, to help prepare for an important class or exam at school, or to center themselves before an important game or event.

Once, after a progressive relaxation session with a teenage patient experiencing extreme pain, the patient's father told the hospital pain-management team I was the magic pill that made his son feel better. I am not a magic pill. I did nothing more than guide this young man to something that was there all along. The ability to slow down the breath and progressively relax his body, to mindfully respond to pain in a reflective rather than a reflexive way, existed within him. I merely showed him how to find it.

Grateful parents have quietly whispered to me, *"How did you do that?"* as their child, previously inconsolable and uncomfortable, finally relaxed into a restful sleep. One teenage boy, recovering from hip surgery, claimed the guided meditation I offered him was "stupid awesome!" I agree. Meditation *is* stupid awesome. But it's also very simple. So simple, in fact, it's child's play.

This book is divided into five sections, based on each activity's focus area, allowing you to quickly navigate to techniques that meet your child's needs, be it pain control, letting off steam, deep relaxation, focusing before a test, or energizing when bogged down by a midafternoon slump. The parts include:

- I'M THE BOSS OF MY BREATH. Techniques that use the breath as a tool to self-regulate and meditate.

- HOCUS POCUS, I CAN FOCUS. Activities to clear the mind and focus on the present moment and task at hand.

- STRESS BUSTERS AND ENERGY EQUALIZERS. Activities to develop kids' self-awareness and teach them how to recognize and manage states of excess energy, depleted energy, or stress within the body.

- **THE CHILL ZONE.** Techniques to disconnect, chill out, and relax.
- **CONNECT.** Games to play with friends or classmates that deliver the benefits of breath control and meditation along with a whole lot of fun!

Many techniques cross over between sections and serve double or triple duty—for example, an exercise that appears in the mind-focused part "Hocus Pocus, I Can Focus" may very well be an effective tool to unplug and relax or access the breath to calm and center oneself. This book features active and passive meditation exercises. Active meditations usually involve movement and/or play; such exercises are helpful for kids and beginners learning to meditate as well as those who may find sitting still especially challenging. Passive meditations tend to require a little more stillness and inner reflection and may be incrementally introduced as your child's skills strengthen.

I recommend using this book as a guide to encourage your kids to explore the mind–body connection and discover which activities they enjoy and find most helpful. Involve them as much as you can, particularly in discussions after practice about how they feel and how they may apply what they learned to different situations in their lives. Self-inquiry evolves to self-awareness and ultimately self-care.

Working with and caring for children, we share a common desire to enrich their lives by providing solid, stable foundations to build happy, successful, and healthy futures. If you work with children, or have children in your life, this book is for you . . . and for *them*.

- Lisa Roberts

Getting Started

E ach technique in this book is presented in a fun, kid-friendly format, focusing on a few straightforward questions: *What is it? How does it help? What do you need?* These questions are followed by "Simple Steps for Kids"—easy-to-follow instructions you can read directly to your children, which they can follow and practice, regardless of meditation experience or age. If your child can read, she should be able to follow the instructions. And if your little one is not yet a reader, you will be able to easily guide him through the exercises. Exploring the breath and mind–body connection is enjoyable for kids and adults alike; you will benefit from these techniques as much as your child does, and, most importantly, you will be connecting with your child in a beneficial and playful way. Before beginning the exercises, there are a few easy instructions to keep in mind.

GUIDELINES

If props are required for an activity, they will be listed before the instructions, along with suggestions for alternative props should you not have access to those suggested. To ensure comfort and safety, the basic posture guide on page 8 provides suggestions for seated, standing, and supine postures when practicing the games and techniques presented in this book.

As you and your children (or students) perform the various activities, your role is to guide them as they explore the breath and mind–body connection and encourage them to observe how they feel after practicing the techniques. Through practice and reflection, kids begin to recognize how each technique helps them and will be empowered to access it whenever they may need it!

The most important instructions for using this book are to jump right in and try all of the exercises, have fun, and discover what works best for the children in your life.

Working with Younger Children

Young kids can be a little overzealous when first learning breathing techniques. Be wary of this and encourage them to develop stable and controlled breathing patterns. I recommend introducing breath regulation through games and play, practicing for short periods, and allowing plenty of "normal breathing" breaks in between.

The beauty of these exercises is that you do not need to explain why you are doing them; simply jump right in and guide younger children by practicing the technique with them. *Play*, don't teach: Make it fun and they will benefit! End each practice with an open discussion—acknowledge any differences they noticed in the way they breathed and how these changes made them feel.

Younger children may not make a conscious connection between their breath and their minds or bodies, yet subconsciously they will come to understand the way they breathe while playing the games or practicing the exercises helps them to feel better and more relaxed.

Working with Older Children and Teens

Older children are curious to learn what each technique is and how it specifically helps them. The simple format allows for easy explanation and a handy way to share the information so that kids can refer back to it any time they need it.

As with younger children, encourage an open discussion after practice and explore how each activity made them feel. Encourage kids to think about where they may apply these skills and practices in their lives.

While it may elicit moans and groans, it is important to have the kids disconnect from their electronic devices while practicing these techniques. Switch off all cell phones and gadgets and put them aside before beginning. In extreme cases, such as hospitalized patients who may need to keep their phones on so family can reach them, phones may be switched to vibrate mode and kept nearby. Be judicious and be sure to convey the benefits of disconnecting to your children or students.

A Word of Caution

The meditation activities in this book are all simple and fun, but there are still some precautions to keep in mind:

- The breath should never be forced. Even when an exercise calls for deep breathing, it should feel natural, with steady and evenly controlled breaths. If the breath becomes choppy or strained, stop practicing immediately and return to normal breathing.

- Slowly increase the number of rounds and/or practice time for each exercise incrementally and approach each practice anew. No matter how long you and your child practiced during a previous session, always begin slowly and build up to your comfort level.

- Short breaks to return to normal breath are encouraged, especially when first working with breathing techniques.

- Correct posture is vital. It creates the space within the body needed to access the respiratory system and allows one to be more comfortable while practicing. Using correct posture while meditating will improve one's general posture, positively affecting the skeletal, muscular, digestive, and circulatory systems and increasing self-esteem.

Handy-Dandy Tips

Here are even more ways for you and your child to get more out of meditation:

- Some techniques will guide you to "scan your body." This simply means to slowly and carefully check in with the entire body from the top of the head, all the way to the toes, and notice how each part of the body feels. Is your child holding on to tension somewhere—clenching his jaw, squeezing his fingers or toes, or shrugging his shoulders? Sometimes your child will be cued to scan after a technique to see how different he feels and whether the technique has helped him. (For a whole exercise on this technique, see Body Scan on page 138.)

- Music can be incorporated to add to the ambience and encourage deeper levels of relaxation. Ambient music can be found online or at music and health stores.

- Set the mood for relaxation by reducing harsh light and drawing the shades where possible. Do not make it completely dark, as this may be frightening for some children.

- Complementary therapies may be included, where appropriate, to enhance the experience. Aromatherapy, reflexology, and massage are some suggestions worth exploring.

- Journaling or crafting is encouraged, especially following meditation and relaxation exercises. This allows children to explore their inner consciousness and the effects the practice has on their mind and body. Journaling can also be enlightening for parents and teachers.

- Most techniques are adaptable for all ages. Use discretion and adapt the activity to the developmental age of your children.

- Generally, the techniques do not need to be practiced in a specific or ideal place. Use discretion, yet be creative and teach kids how to access these techniques anywhere and anytime the need arises—for example, while waiting in long lines at the movies or amusement park, or before a test.

- Keep a box of tissues on hand, as sinuses can be stimulated when practicing breathing techniques and tissues may be needed to help clear them out. Be sure to tell the children this may happen and give them permission to help themselves to the tissue box as needed.

- A child may fall asleep during relaxation, or may need to go to the bathroom. Give permission before commencing activities so the child feels safe and comfortable if she drifts off to sleep, or, if she needs to leave the room to go to the bathroom, she can do so without disrupting others.

- If a child falls asleep and you need to wake him, do so gently. A feather is a gentle way to wake a child—be sure to explain to your kids this is how you will wake them if they fall asleep *before* practicing, so they are not surprised and jolted out of their chilled out, relaxed space.

POSTURE GUIDE FOR YOU AND YOUR CHILD

Poor posture leads to an unhealthy muscular and skeletal system, and can negatively impact circulation, digestion, breathing, and self-esteem. When practicing meditation, kids need access to their full breathing system—nose, mouth, throat, lungs, diaphragm, chest, back, and belly. If you were slouching in a chair, or curled in a ball on the sofa, do you think your body position would allow access to all of those areas, giving you enough space to breath naturally and freely? No way!

Good posture allows access to our full breathing apparatus while practicing breathing techniques. With time and practice, your kid's general posture will naturally improve, creating space in the body for better breathing on a daily basis, along with a host of additional health benefits. It is also important for kids to feel comfortable, supported, and relaxed while practicing meditation, eliminating physical strain, which only adds to or creates tension.

The following guide demonstrates postures recommended for seated, standing, or supine practice, along with the recommended use of bolsters, blankets, and props to ensure comfort and support no matter how you and your child choose to practice.

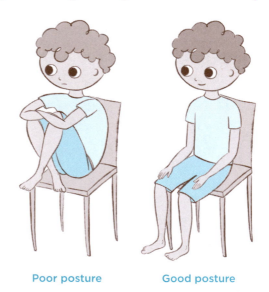

Poor posture   Good posture

Crisscross

- Sit crisscross with one ankle in front of the other on the floor or on a yoga mat.

- Allow knees to fall out to the sides.

- Rest hands on the thighs and be sure the shoulders are relaxed—imagine both shoulder blades sliding down your back as the shoulders relax away from the ears.

- Gently press the sit bones into the floor and feel the spine float to an erect position as you do so. This should feel natural and not forced; the spine and body should be upright but not rigid.

- Keep the chin level with the floor.

- Scan the body and be sure you are not holding tension anywhere while maintaining this posture. Remain erect yet relaxed.

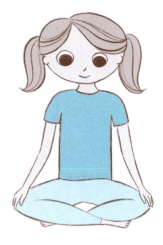

Crisscross

Adjustments

- Placing a folded-up blanket, yoga block, cushion, or pillow under the butt helps support the spine, hips, and knees in this position. It can also be more comfortable on your tush!

- Additional support can be added under the knees where needed, using blocks, bolsters, or folded blankets.

TIP: *When sitting crisscross, kids can switch which leg is in front each time they sit. They will gravitate toward their dominant side, but switching legs can help maintain balance in the hips and strengthen the nondominant side.*

Kneeling

- Kneel on the floor or yoga mat, sitting on your heels, hands resting on the thighs.

- Be sure the shoulders are relaxed: Imagine both shoulder blades sliding down your back as the shoulders relax away from the ears.

- The chin should be level and the spine naturally erect, with the spine and body upright but not rigid.

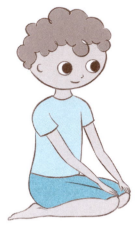

Kneeling

Adjustment

If this position puts too much strain on the knees, do not sit on your heels. Instead, place a yoga block or bolster between the calves and sit on it. You will still be kneeling, but your butt will rest on the prop, placing less stress on the knees.

TIP: *If kids find they are slouching or are having trouble sitting up straight in any of the floor-seated postures, they can try sitting against a wall or using a chair.*

SEATED AGAINST A WALL

Find a clear wall space, without anything on it such as artwork or shelving.

- Place a folded blanket or bolster on the floor and against the wall to sit on. Once seated, walk the butt back to make contact with the wall.

- Crisscross the legs with one ankle in front of the other. If this is difficult or uncomfortable, sit with the legs extended straight out.

- Relax the back against the wall, allowing it to support the torso.

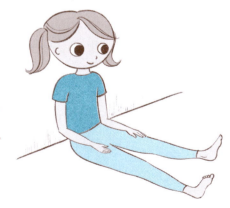

Against wall

- Rest your hands in your lap and relax the shoulders—imagine both shoulder blades sliding down your back as the shoulders relax away from the ears.

- Gently press the sit bones into the floor or bolster and feel the spine grow tall; this should feel natural and not forced.

- Keeping the chin level with the floor, remain relaxed and allow the wall to help support you.

Adjustment

Place a pillow, bolster, or folded blanket between the lumbar spine and the wall where needed for extra support.

SEATED ON CHAIR

You will need a sturdy chair with a straight back for support.

- Sit on the chair with both feet planted firmly on the floor in front of it. You may need to scoot forward on the chair in order to reach the floor comfortably with both feet. Consider a smaller, kid-size chair for your child, so that his feet can reach the ground.

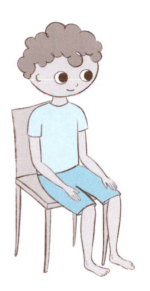

On chair

- Rest hands on the thighs and be sure the shoulders are relaxed—imagine both shoulder blades sliding down your back as the shoulders relax away from the ears.

- Gently press the sit bones into the chair and feel the spine float to an erect position as you do so. This should feel natural and not forced.

- Keep the chin level with the floor.

- Scan the body and be sure you are not holding tension anywhere while maintaining this posture.

- Remain erect yet relaxed, keeping the spine and body upright, but not rigid.

Adjustment

If the lumbar support or back of the chair does not support your back—which may happen when both feet are on the floor—then place a pillow, bolster, or blanket between the back of the chair and the torso for additional support.

STANDING

When practicing breathing or relaxation techniques while standing, make sure to stand solid, strong, and still, like a mountain. Build your mountain like this:

- Begin standing with feet hip-width distance apart.

- Press both feet evenly into the floor and feel the sternum slightly pull up as the spine floats to a naturally erect position.

- Rest the arms alongside the torso and be sure the shoulders are relaxed—imagine both shoulder blades sliding down your back as the shoulders relax away from the ears.

- Place your palms face forward with the fingers spread like stars.

- Allow the chin to be level with the floor.

- Scan the body and be sure you are not holding tension anywhere while maintaining this posture. Remain upright yet relaxed and not rigid . . . just like a mountain!

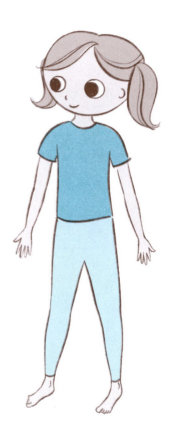

Mountain

SUPINE

The supine posture and adjustments described below are for practice while lying on a yoga mat or the floor; they can be adapted for use on a bed or sofa where necessary.

- Begin by lying on the floor.

- Hug the knees into the chest and feel the spine flatten along the floor.

- Release the legs, one at a time, stretching them out along the floor.

- Allow the feet to fall open, relaxed.

- Tuck the shoulder blades under one at a time—this opens the chest and front side of the torso—and then relax the shoulders and upper body on the floor.

- Allow the arms to rest on the floor alongside the torso.

- Rest hands with the palms facing up, or else fold them in and rest palms down on the belly.

- Let go of any muscle engagement and allow the floor to fully support the body.

Adjustments

- Support and protect the lower back by placing a pillow, rolled-up blanket, or bolster just below the knees. Or, bend the knees so they point toward the ceiling and place the feet flat on the floor, a few inches from the hips and hip-width distance apart. Knees can fall in, resting against one another, or remain separated.

- Support the head and neck by using a pillow or folded-up blanket under the head.

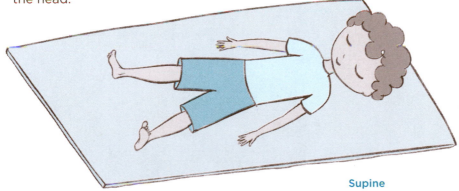

Supine

I'm the Boss of My Breath

ALL ABOUT:
BREATHING TECHNIQUES FOR CALM, STILL, IN-CONTROL KIDS

Breathing is a pretty simple yet vital function that occurs involuntarily—that is, without effort or thought. Unfortunately, we humans are inherently lazy and don't use our entire breathing apparatus to breathe fully. Getting by on short, shallow breaths, many people do not know how to breathe well and are unaware that it is possible to take control of the breath and, ultimately, how we feel. This section features fun games and tools that teach kids breath awareness and proper breathing techniques. The benefits of practicing breathing techniques include self-regulation (the ability to regulate mood and excitement levels), improved posture, enhanced mental clarity and ability to focus, increased blood circulation and oxygen levels, and effective pain control.

Sounds Great . . . but How Do I Convey This to My Kids?

Use play and discussion! Play around with the techniques in this chapter and see which ones resonate with the kids you are working with. Encourage post-practice discussion—without leading—focusing on how they felt while practicing each technique. It is empowering for kids to realize they can access these techniques on their own, any time they need them.

Why Breathing? Isn't This Book about Meditation?

It is! Meditation may not be easy, but it *is* simple. The breath is a wonderful tool to access when learning to establish present-moment awareness. Providing a strong anchor to focus on, the breath keeps one connected to each moment as it unfolds. This is meditation.

Guidelines

As you and your child are practicing with the breath, keep in mind:

- Breath work should always be approached with a sense of ease and gentleness.

- If feelings of discomfort or shortness of breath are experienced, STOP practicing immediately and recommence regular breathing.

- Never force the breath or create tension within the body.

- Forget how many rounds you completed or how long you practiced yesterday. Approach each practice as if you were doing the exercise for the first time. Start slow and incrementally build to your child's comfort level.

- Be very mindful to convey these guidelines to children who tend to be a little overzealous when initially learning breathing exercises. Foster an understanding of *doing* without *trying* and revert to activities such as Bubble Breath (page 24) or Bubbles in Milk (page 26) to demonstrate the sensation of elongating and smoothing the breath without forcing it.

STRESS TEST

What Is Stress Test and How Does It Help?

In moments of stress or anxiety we often hold our breath and tense up our bodies without even realizing it. Stress Test demonstrates this phenomenon in action, teaching us to be aware of this response and how we can change it by consciously relaxing our bodies and taking control of our breath. This exercise gives kids an important message: *You are the boss of your breath!* No matter what is happening, you have the ability to step in and take control. Let's try it!

» *Also good for: stress-busting*

What Do You Need?

You will need any one of the following:

- A soft rubber or fabric stress ball
- A wad of balled-up tissue paper
- A pair of balled-up socks

No Props? No Problem!

Have kids tense up their fists and squeeze them as tightly as they can for a count of ten.

SIMPLE STEPS FOR KIDS

- Squeeze a prop from the list above in your fist as tightly as you can for ten seconds. Squeeze really, really tightly for the whole ten seconds!

- What happens to your breath? Your shoulders? Other areas of your body?

- Now repeat the first step, but consciously breathe slowly and deeply as you squeeze the prop.

- Scan your body and relax any areas, other than the fist squeezing the prop, where you are tensing up.

- Can you squeeze the prop as tightly as possible while breathing deeply *and* consciously relaxing the rest of your body? It takes a little effort, but it is possible.

- Notice how different this feels from the first try, when you most likely held your breath and tensed up your entire body.

HOBERMAN SPHERE

What Is a Hoberman Sphere?

A Hoberman sphere is a plastic, dome-shaped toy with a hinge-like joint action that allows it to fold down to a small, compact ball and expand out to a large sphere shape.

How Does It Help?

A Hoberman sphere can be used as a visual tool to help kids connect to their breath by observing it. Our lungs are very similar to a Hoberman sphere in that they expand when we inhale and relax when we exhale. Linking the simple expansion and relaxation of the Hoberman sphere to our own inhales and exhales serves as a visual aid to observe the breath, enabling kids to work toward slowing and deepening the breath as well as learning how to "even it out"—inhaling and exhaling smoothly and for an equal count.

» *Also good for: focus*

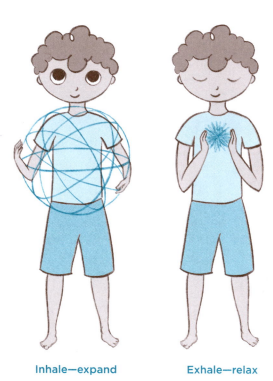

Inhale—expand   Exhale—relax

TIP: *Once your child has mastered evening out his inhales and exhales, and feels comfortable with this type of breathing (i.e., it feels natural and not forced), he can challenge himself by learning to extend the exhale—that is, making the exhale last a little longer than the inhale. Build slowly, incrementally making your exhale longer and longer, but never make the exhale last longer than two times the inhale.*

SIMPLE STEPS FOR KIDS

- Begin in a comfortable seated position, sitting tall but relaxed.
- As you breathe in, slowly expand the Hoberman sphere for the duration of your inhale. Once your inhale is complete, stop expanding the sphere.
- Notice the natural pause between your inhale and exhale.
- As you begin to exhale, collapse the Hoberman sphere until your exhale is complete. Stop and notice the natural pause before your inhale begins. Repeat.
- Notice how far you expand the sphere as you inhale. Does the sphere move all the way back to the same starting point when you complete your exhale? If not, work toward making the movement of the Hoberman sphere—and your inhale and exhale—even.

No Hoberman Sphere? No Problem!

Kids can use their hands if they do not have access to a Hoberman sphere! Just give them the following instructions: Begin with the palms pressed together in front of your torso. Breathe in, slowly moving the palms away from one another and stopping when you complete your inhale. Notice the natural pause between your inhale and exhale. As you exhale, slowly move the palms back to meet each other. Was your inhale as long as your exhale? Did your hands meet back together at the end of your exhale? Work toward making this happen.

PINWHEEL BREATHING

What Is Pinwheel Breathing?

We all have the power and strength of the wind within us. Kids prove it when they play with pinwheels! Blowing hard, they make them spin wild and fast, but can they make them spin slowly and steadily for a long time? Of course they can!

How Does It Help?

Pinwheels are a fun way to explore the breath and how we can control it to benefit our mind and our body. By playing with pinwheels, kids teach themselves to extend the out breath (exhale) and discover how this can lead to feelings of relaxation.

» *Also good for: stress-busting*

What Do You Need?

- A pinwheel. You can buy these at a dollar store or, if you are feeling creative, you can make one (you can find tutorials at various craft websites).

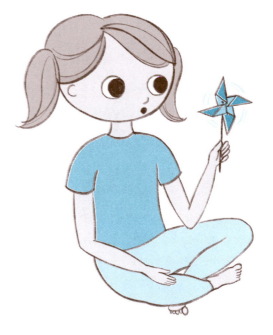

Exhale

SIMPLE STEPS FOR KIDS

- Begin in a comfortable seated position.

- Take a deep breath in through the nose and bring the pinwheel a few inches from your mouth.

- Gently exhale, blowing the pinwheel so it moves.

- How fast did your pinwheel move? How long did it spin for?

- Take another breath in and blow on your pinwheel again. Can you make your exhale last for a long time so your pinwheel spins even longer than last time?

- Play around with your breath and make your pinwheel spin at different speeds.

- Notice how your body feels when you make the pinwheel spin for a long time versus when you make it spin fast.

- Notice which parts of your body are active when you change the way you breathe.

- Which breath makes you feel calm and relaxed?

BUBBLE BREATH

What Is Bubble Breath?

Bubble Breath is a fun way to explore the breath and how it can help kids relax and feel good.

How Does It Help?

Providing a great visual, Bubble Breath is an excellent way for kids to learn about their breath by physically seeing what happens when they breathe differently. As they play, they will learn what type of breathing makes them feel better and more relaxed. And who doesn't want to have fun while learning?

» *Also good for: stress-busting*

What Do You Need?

- Bubble wand
- Liquid soap

TIP:

- *For extra fun, try colored bubbles or special bubbles that don't pop easily.*
- *Bubbles can leave a sticky residue on the floor or create a slippery mess. Encourage your child to blow bubbles in an area where nothing will get damaged and that is safe, such as outside with adult supervision.*

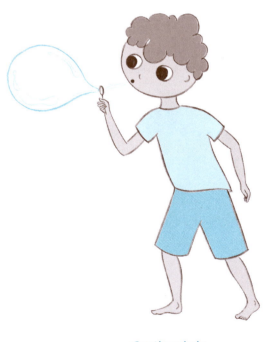

Gentle exhale

SIMPLE STEPS FOR KIDS

- Swirl your bubble wand in liquid soap and then hold it a few inches from your lips.

- Gently blow through pursed lips as you watch your bubble grow.

- Try blowing a sharp burst of air through the wand. Can you make a bubble this way?

- Which works better: a long, gentle, steady stream of air, or a short, powerful burst?

- Notice how these two different breaths make you feel. Which parts of your body engage or relax with each breath?

- Which breath feels easier? Does one require less effort?

- Which breath makes the biggest bubbles?

- Have fun! Make as many big, beautiful bubbles as you can.

- Feel good! Notice how slowly blowing bubbles makes you feel super relaxed.

BUBBLES IN MILK

What Is Bubbles in Milk?

Bubbles in Milk is a fun way for kids to learn about the breath. Kids of all ages love this—even big kids (especially those who, like me, were told not to do this as a child!).

How Does It Help?

Blowing bubbles in milk creates a strong visual, allowing kids to see when long, controlled exhales are at work and when they are not, as well as what effect each creates—milk splashing and spilling everywhere, or a nice controlled pile of bubbles building up. An activity that is fun and educational—what more could you ask for?

» *Also good for: stress-busting*

What Do You Need?

- Plastic cup
- Straw
- Milk (almond milk bubbles up very well)

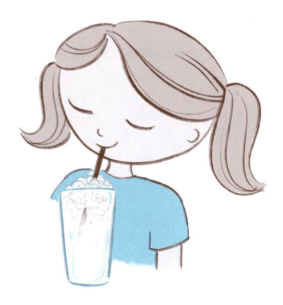

Slow exhale

SIMPLE STEPS FOR KIDS

- Fill the plastic cup a little less than halfway with milk.

- Place the straw in the cup.

- Take a full breath in through your nose and, once you have completed your inhale, place the straw in your mouth, gently pursing your lips around it.

- Slowly exhale through the straw and watch the bubbles form.

- The best way to make lots of bubbles is to blow into the straw very slowly for as long as possible.

- Play around with this exercise. Blow hard and see the difference in the type of bubbles this creates. Notice how quickly the bubbles dissipate. Do you notice any difference between those created with long, slow exhales and those made with short, sharp bursts of air?

SINGING BREATH

What Is Singing Breath and How Does It Help?

Singing Breath is a fun way for kids to make some noise and release tension. It also helps bring awareness to the breath, teaching kids to breathe fully and deeply, which promotes relaxation.

» *Also good for: stress-busting*

SIMPLE STEPS FOR KIDS

We will use the vowel sounds of the alphabet (*A-E-I-O-U*) to describe this exercise, but you can use any sounds at all! Feel free to sing your name or the name of a friend, or even something as simple as *do, re, mi.* The only rules are to have fun and to use the entire out breath (or exhale) to make your sound.

- Take a big breath in, filling up your lungs. Sweep your arms up overhead as you breathe in; this allows more space for the ribs to expand, resulting in a fuller "in breath" or inhale.

- Open your mouth and exhale by singing the letter *A* until all of the air is out of your body—like this: "Aaaaaaaa . . . " The sound should stop once you have emptied all the air from your lungs. Float the arms back down by your sides as you sing the sound.

- Take another deep breath in, sweeping the arms up overhead, and repeat with the next vowel—"Eeeeeeee . . . "—and so on.

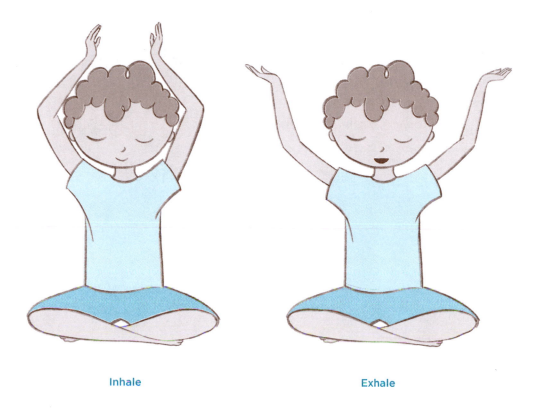

Inhale

Exhale

TIP: *Kids should not be afraid to make noise or laugh. Making noise and laughing are great ways to release tension from the body!*

FEATHER BREATH

What Is Feather Breath?

Feather Breath utilizes fun games and colorful feathers to teach more about how we breathe and how we can change our breath in order to feel more relaxed or energized.

» *Also good for: focus*

What Do You Need?

- Feathers
- Straws

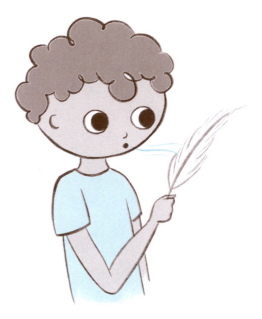

See your breath

 SIMPLE STEPS FOR KIDS

SEEING THE BREATH

- Rest a single feather in the open palm of your hand, holding it just below the chin.
- Breathe normally.
- Watch the feather closely and notice how it responds. Can you tell which is your inhale and which is your exhale based on the movement of the feather?

EXHALING

Now that you know what your breath looks like and that you can move the feather when you are breathing normally, let's explore how exhaling can feel different, not only for the feather but for you!

- Hold the feather upright, placing the stem between your thumb and index finger.

- Notice how the feather has soft, light plumes, while other parts of the feather are stiff.

- Use your breath to move only the soft parts of the feather.

- Now use the breath to move the stiffer parts.

- What do you notice about the way you must exhale to move the soft parts of the feather? And the stiff? How does each exhale make you feel?

- Play around some more and notice which parts of your body move when making the different breaths. Where does the breath originate? Which body parts relax or contract?

- Which exhale makes you feel good?

FEATHER STORM

Not unlike autumn leaf storms, feather storms are fun to play in with your friends. You will need two or more people, one straw for each person, and a small (or large) pile of feathers to place on the floor between you.

- Lie on your bellies on the floor with the feathers scattered in the middle.

- Blow through the straws, aiming at the feathers to make them rise up and swirl around.

- Can you keep the storm blowing? Can you work together to make sure none of the feathers fly outside the circle?

- Does one type of exhale help you play this game better? If so, which one?

FEATHER FLOAT

To play Feather Float you will need a straw and a feather.

- Toss the feather high up in the air and blow through the straw to keep the feather off the ground.

- If playing in a group, the person who keeps the feather from hitting the ground longest is the winner.

- If playing individually, time yourself and keep trying to beat your own time by keeping the feather in the air as long as you can.

- What kind of exhale helps you play this game better?

FEATHER PASS

To play Feather Pass you will need a minimum of two players and one feather per group.

- Sit facing your partner if in pairs, or in a small circle if in groups.

- Rest a feather in the palm of the hand and gently blow on it until it floats through the air to your partner. (If in a group, the player with the feather chooses which person they blow the feather to and so on).

- Your partner must try to catch the feather and pass it back to you or to another player.

- Notice the breath. How must you breathe to control the direction the feather floats?

SNORKEL BREATH

What Is Snorkel Breath and How Does It Help?

Similar to a pipe or straw, a snorkel enables swimmers to keep their faces submerged in the water, so they can observe fish, coral, and sea life, and breathe at the same time. Snorkel Breath is a technique that uses a straw to emphasize a full exhale, triggering a naturally occurring deeper inhale.

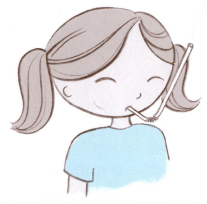

Snorkeling

What Do You Need?

- A regular drinking straw (not a supersize smoothie straw)

TIP: *Bendy straws are fun to use as they can be curved into the shape of a snorkel.*

SIMPLE STEPS FOR KIDS

- Take a full breath in through your nose. Then place the straw in your mouth, gently pursing your lips around it.

- Slowly exhale through the straw.

- Once your exhale is complete, remove the straw and breathe normally for a couple of cycles before repeating.

- Practice Snorkel Breath for a few rounds, building on the number of cycles you complete each time you practice.

- Try a game! Scatter images of sea creatures on the floor. Breathe in, put on your "snorkel", breathe out, and pick a random sea creature. Remove snorkel and create a shape with your body based on your "catch."

ELEVATOR RIDE

What Is Elevator Ride?

Elevator Ride is a breathing technique that uses creative visualization to teach deep-breathing skills while promoting excellent posture.

How Does It Help?

Focusing on the spine and the breath together in this exercise encourages the improvement of general posture. Good posture is healthy for kids' skeletal and muscular systems, and creates space in the torso for better-quality and deeper breathing on a daily basis. Visualizing the breath as a moving object is helpful in slowing down the breath, aiding relaxation.

» *Also good for: focus*

TIP: *Remind your child to breathe smoothly and evenly! If his breath truly were powering an elevator, it would be his job to control the breath to ensure those riding inside enjoy a safe and stable ride!*

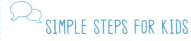 SIMPLE STEPS FOR KIDS

- Begin in a comfortable seated position, either crisscross or kneeling with your butt resting on your heels. Use props as needed for support and comfort.

- Rest your hands on top of your thighs and gently close your eyes. Be sure the shoulders are relaxed.

- Gently press your sit bones down, allowing the spine to float to a naturally erect position.

- Visualize your spine running from your tailbone all the way to your skull. Now imagine that your spine is an elevator shaft, with an elevator cab that travels up and down your spine.

- As you breathe in, feel the elevator rise from your tailbone, all the way to the top floor—your head. Feel the spine grow light and tall as the elevator rises on your inhale.

- As you breathe out, feel the elevator travel back down the spine, all the way to the basement—your tailbone. Feel grounded and stable as the elevator lowers on your exhale. Imagine it taking any unwanted feelings, worries, or concerns with it as it lowers. Imagine these feelings getting off the elevator before your next inhale.

- Continue with elevator breath for three to five minutes. Return to normal breathing but remain sitting with your eyes closed for a few more minutes. Notice how centered and relaxed you feel.

BELLY BREATHING

What Is Belly Breathing?

Belly Breathing, or diaphragmatic breathing, is a deep-breathing technique used to relax the mind and body, easing physical and mental tension or stress.

» *Also good for: stress-busting, focus, and relaxation*

 ## SIMPLE STEPS FOR KIDS

- Lie in a comfortable position on your yoga mat. As you slowly breathe in, be conscious of filling your lungs all the way. When the lungs expand to capacity, the belly will rise.

- As you breathe out, be sure to fully empty your lungs. Pull your belly button all the way in, as if it could touch your spine! (This won't really happen, but it is a good visual to help you fully expel all of the air.)

- Repeat for several rounds, until you feel calm and relaxed.

Belly Breathing may feel weird at first, especially if you are not used to breathing slowly and deeply, or focusing your attention on your breath. With practice it will get easier and feel less strange, and once you enjoy the benefits, it will become natural to begin Belly Breathing any time you need to relax your mind or body.

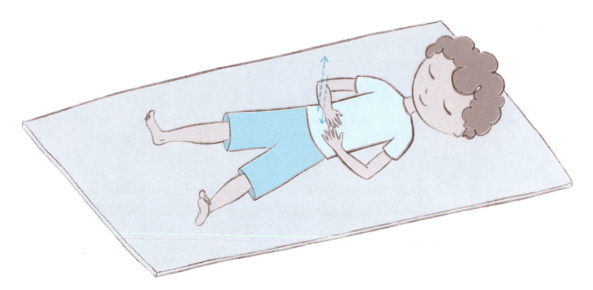

Belly rises and falls with the breath

TIP: *Help your child with a visual! Place her hands, a beanbag, a book, or even a toy (such as a rubber ducky) on her belly to help her observe the effects of deep Belly Breathing.*

BACK BREATHING

What Is Back Breathing?

Back Breathing is exactly as it sounds: a breathing technique where the focus is on directing the breath into the back area of the body.

How Does It Help?

When we breathe in, our chest expands to accommodate the expansion of the lungs as they fill with air. The problem is, we usually do not breathe as fully or deeply as we have the capacity to and the chest barely moves! This technique explores breathing fully and deeply by expanding the chest in all directions, allowing the lungs to take in more oxygen. Have your child try it for a few minutes several times a day and notice how different he feels!

 SIMPLE STEPS FOR KIDS

- Begin in a comfortable seated position, spine naturally erect. If you are sitting on a chair, both feet should be in contact with the floor. Relax the shoulders and allow your hands to rest in your lap.

- Close your eyes and begin to reflect inwardly—that is, let go of what is happening around you and focus on your body and mind.

- Begin to observe the breath. Don't change it; simply notice as you naturally breathe in and out.

- When you feel ready, slowly begin to deepen the breath.

- After a few rounds of deep breathing, direct your focus to your back.

- On your next inhale, visualize the breath "filling up" your entire back. Continue breathing this way for several rounds, noticing how the back spreads and expands with each inhale and relaxes with each exhale. Imagine your shoulder blades spreading like giant wings as you inhale and relaxing as you exhale.

- Return to natural breathing and gently open your eyes. Notice how your body and mind feel.

- For variety, try this exercise sitting with your back against a wall. Feel the back expand and press into the wall as you inhale and relax away from it as you exhale.

PARTNER FUN!

Sit back-to-back with a friend and begin to practice Back Breathing. See if you can feel each other breathe through your backs. Synchronize your breath with your partner's breath; then try alternating breaths with your partner. Notice how different each practice feels.

SIDE BREATHING

What Is Side Breathing?

Side Breathing is a technique where the focus is on directing the breath into the side areas of the torso.

How Does It Help?

As mentioned in Back Breathing (page 38), as we breathe in, the chest is designed to expand in all directions to accommodate the expansion of the lungs as they fill with air. Unfortunately, we're not used to breathing as fully or as deeply as we're able to. Side Breathing is another fun way of teaching kids to do just that! Combined with the Belly Breathing (page 36) and Back Breathing techniques, Side Breathing demonstrates how different it feels to take full, deep breaths. Have your kids try it for a few minutes several times a day and notice how good they feel!

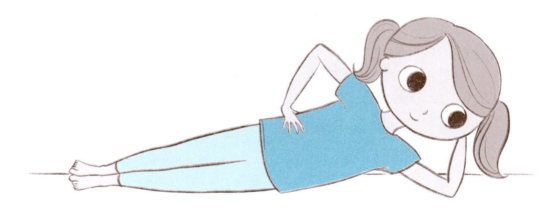

Feel your ribs move with each breath

SIMPLE STEPS FOR KIDS

- Lie on your side and prop your head on a pillow or on a bent elbow or hand.

- Place your other hand on the outer ribs that are facing the ceiling. Gently clasp the outer rib cage between your thumb and fingers.

- Begin breathing deeply, until you feel the ribs expanding into the grip of your hand.

- Exhale and observe the ribs retract under your hand.

- Breathe deeply for several rounds; then flip and try this technique on your other side.

- Once finished, relax for a few moments and notice how you feel.

- Are you naturally breathing more deeply than you were before you tried this exercise?

SANDBAG

What Is Sandbag?

This breathing technique uses a sandbag to encourage the body to exhale fully, promoting a deeper sense of relaxation.

How Does It Help?

Sandbag is a restorative technique, meaning there is very little muscle engagement or effort required to practice. The extra weight of the sandbag on the belly helps kids deepen and slow the breath, and provides sensory input to calm the nervous system—a gentle reminder that it is time to calm down and chill out.

» *Also good for: relaxation*

What Do You Need?

- A small sandbag (it does not need to be heavy; a small amount of weight is enough to add resistance).

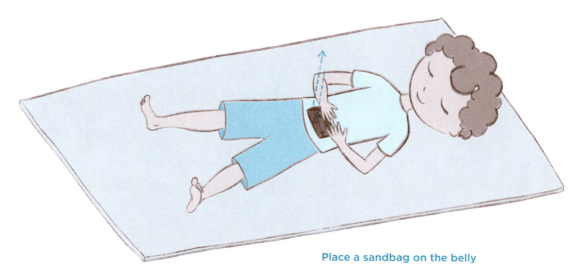

Place a sandbag on the belly

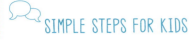

SIMPLE STEPS FOR KIDS

- Begin in a comfortable position resting on your back.

- Allow the feet to fall open and the whole body to relax, fully supported by the floor.

- Place a sandbag on your abdomen and begin to inhale. Notice the resistance as your belly presses against the sandbag.

- Exhale slowly. As you complete your exhale, notice how the weight of the sandbag helps you contract your belly more than usual, allowing a fuller exhale to occur.

- Breathe slowly and deeply for several minutes with the sandbag on your belly.

- Remove the sandbag. Does your breathing pattern change? Are you still exhaling as fully as you did when you felt the slight weight of the sandbag on your belly? Notice how relaxed you feel after just a few minutes of breathing slowly and deeply.

No Sandbag? No Problem!

Use a small bag of sugar, flour, or rice.

THREE-PART BREATH

What Is Three-Part Breath?

Three-Part Breath is a breathing technique that demonstrates how to breathe deeply and fully.

How Does It Help?

Three-Part Breath slows down and steadies your child's breathing, promoting a sense of calm, relaxation, and control. Three-Part Breath teaches kids how to utilize the entire breathing system they were born with, encouraging full and deep inhales rather than the short and shallow breaths people usually get by with.

» *Also good for: focus*

 SIMPLE STEPS FOR KIDS

- Sit comfortably in a chair, spine naturally erect. Your shoulders should be relaxed with hands resting on knees or thighs, and both feet flat on the floor.

- Gently place one hand on the upper chest area below the collarbones and one hand on the belly. Be sure to keep the shoulders and arms relaxed as you rest the hands on these two areas.

- Take a deep, slow breath in through your nose, filling the lower part of your lungs. You should feel your belly pressing against your hand as this happens.

- Slowly breathe out, feeling your belly retract as you do so. Imagine you are pulling your belly button in to touch your spine. This will help fully expel all of the air.

- Breathe in and out this way for five full breaths.

- After five breaths, breathe in once again, this time filling the lungs until the belly presses against your hand. Then sip in a little more air, filling up the chest. Notice the ribs and breastbone expand as the middle of your torso fills with the extra breath.

- As you exhale, feel the ribs relax as the air from your middle releases first, followed by the belly button moving toward the spine as the air expels from the belly.

- Repeat deep breathing into the belly and the rib cage for five full breaths.

- After five breaths, breathe in again, filling up the belly, followed by the rib cage. Then, fill the upper-chest cavity with more air so that you feel your collarbones spreading, almost like they are breaking into a huge smile.

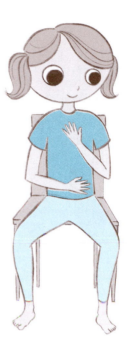

Relax shoulders and elbows

- Exhale, first emptying the upper chest so that the collarbones relax, then the middle chest, and finally the belly. Pulling the belly button all the way toward the spine, fully expel all of the air.

- Continue to breathe this way for five full breaths.

- You are now practicing Three-Part Breath. As you practice, work toward making the three parts one smooth movement rather than breaking them up with pauses. It will still be Three-Part Breath—filling the lower, middle, and upper torso—but in one long breath, without pauses. The exhale will be the same: first emptying the upper torso, then the middle, and, finally, the lower torso, in one long exhale.

- Repeat for five to ten rounds.

EQUAL BREATH

What Is Equal Breath?

Equal Breath is exactly as it sounds—an exercise where kids control their breath by breathing in and out to an equal count.

How Does It Help?

Equal Breath relaxes the body while fully engaging the mind, making it an excellent exercise in concentration or focus. Kids can use this exercise to relax during moments of stress, to refocus before an important class, or to help quiet the mind and relax the body if they are having trouble sleeping.

» *Also good for: focus*

TIP: *Kids will experience the effects of this exercise with a lower count; they will not experience any positive effects from this exercise by forcing a higher count, creating tension in the body and mind. Always have kids check in with their bodies as they practice this exercise. Each time they should approach it as new, build the count slowly, and always drop back to a lower count if they notice any pressure on the body, mind, or breath.*

SIMPLE STEPS FOR KIDS

- Begin in a comfortable position either seated or lying on your back.

- Close your eyes and turn your attention inward.

- Shift your attention to your breath. Do not change anything about your breath; just let it flow in and out naturally, observing it as it does so.

- As you breathe in, count in your mind: 1-2-3.

- As you breathe out, count in your mind: 1-2-3.

- Once you complete several rounds, and breathing this way feels comfortable, increase the count.

- As you breathe in, count in your mind: 1-2-3-4.

- As your breathe out, count in your mind: 1-2-3-4.

- After several rounds, scan the body and see if you are holding tension anywhere. If you still feel relaxed, try adding an extra count for a few rounds (for example, 1-2-3-4-5). If breathing this way has created tension somewhere in your body or mind, then relax and go back to a lower count, such as 1-2-3.

LENGTHENING THE EXHALE

What Is Lengthening the Exhale and How Does It Help?

When we breathe in, we inhale fresh oxygen, which our body needs. Our lungs expand and our diaphragm contracts. When we exhale, our lungs and diaphragm relax. Our bodies physically "let go," releasing converted carbon dioxide gases that the body does not need. Essentially, when we breathe in, we are expanding and filling ourselves up with what we need, and when we breathe out, we are letting go of stuff we don't need or that is no longer useful. Lengthening the Exhale helps kids cultivate a deeper sense of release and relaxation within the body and the mind; it also slows down the breath, which calms the nervous system and relieves feelings of stress or anxiety as well as physical tension.

» *Also good for: focus*

TIP: *This technique provides two helpful anchors to the present moment: observing the breath connects kids to each moment, and counting each inhale and exhale requires additional present-moment awareness. It's virtually impossible to be practicing this technique and thinking about something else!*

SIMPLE STEPS FOR KIDS

- Begin in a comfortable position, either seated on the floor or in a chair, or lying down with the knees bent and feet flat on the floor.

- Shift your focus to your breath. Observe it in its natural state for a few rounds.

- Begin to deepen and slow the breath.

- Count your inhale and your exhale and work toward making them last for the same number of counts. For example, inhale, 1-2-3; exhale, 1-2-3.

- Following several rounds of equal breathing, begin to slow down your exhale even more until it is several counts slower than the inhale. For example, inhale, 1-2-3; exhale, 1-2-3-4.

- Be sure to exhale fully each time before breathing in again.

- *Never* take the inhale-to-exhale ratio beyond 1:2. In other words, never exhale for a count greater than double your inhale count.

- Use your imagination! As you breathe out, visualize letting go of any thoughts or feelings that hold you back—anything from anger to jealousy to self-doubt. Allow these feelings to leave with each exhale.

FOUR-SQUARE BREATHING

What Is Four-Square Breathing?

Breathing is something we do naturally without thinking too much about it. If we were to describe how we breathe, we would most likely say that we breathe in and out in two simple steps. But, there are actually four steps to each breath we take:

1. Inhale
2. Pause
3. Exhale
4. Pause

Four-Square Breathing is a technique used to emphasize each stage of the breath, slowing it down and calming the mind, body, and nervous system.

How Does It Help?

An effective relaxation tool, this technique is extremely helpful in alleviating kids' anxiety and stress. They can use it to center themselves before a test, or in any situation when they want to feel calm and focused.

» *Also good for: focus*

TIP: *As kids practice and become more comfortable with this breathing technique, they should incrementally build up to ten full rounds with a count of four for each stage: Inhale for four, hold in for four, exhale for four, and hold out for four. They should* never *go higher than four counts for each stage of the breath. Remind them to take their time and* build slowly *to this level when their* body *is ready (not their mind).*

SIMPLE STEPS FOR KIDS

- Begin in a comfortable seated position, spine naturally erect and chin level. Be sure that your shoulders, arms, and face are relaxed. Hands should rest comfortably in your lap or on your knees.

- Observe your breath's natural cycle for a few rounds before beginning to deepen it.

- Breathe all the way in until your belly expands, and then all the way out until the belly button moves toward the spine, expelling all of the air.

- When you feel ready to begin, inhale to a count of three.

- Once the inhale is complete, hold the breath in for a count of two.

- Slowly exhale for a count of three.

- Hold all of the air out for a count of two.

- Continue breathing this way for three to five full rounds.

OCEAN BREATH

What Is Ocean Breath?

Ocean Breath is a loud, rhythmic breathing technique that really does sound like the ocean. Connecting to the sound and rhythm of the breath using this method has two advantages: The breath can be used as a focal point in meditation to direct kids' minds to the present moment. It can also be used as a gauge during physical activity. When we overstress the body, the breath becomes choppy or strained, serving as a sign that kids should scale back whatever they are doing until the breath sounds smooth, even, and unstressed once again.

How Does It Help?

Focusing on the breath and the sound it creates improves concentration and calms and focuses the mind. This technique is effective for calming the nervous system, reducing pain, and helping with insomnia and headaches.

» *Also good for: focus*

TIP: *When children practice this technique they naturally slow down their breath, making this exercise a great go-to tool to deactivate stress responses anytime and anyplace. (This is true for adults too, of course!)*

SIMPLE STEPS FOR KIDS

- Begin in a comfortable seated position. Sit up tall yet relaxed.

- Take a slow inhale through the nose.

- Open the mouth and exhale with an "ah" sound.

- Repeat two or three times.

- Inhale through the nose; then exhale as if making the "ah" sound without opening your mouth.

- You should hear your breath make a soft "hissing" sound like the ocean.

- Continue to breathe this way, in and out through the nose with your mouth closed, making the gentle hissing sound as if you were breathing out of the mouth saying "ah."

- Keep breathing this way for several rounds. You may notice that your throat constricts slightly to create this rhythmic sound. While this is normal, make sure the breath remains smooth and controlled, and not strained or forced.

- Build up slowly, taking breaks in between to breathe naturally. At first this technique may feel weird, but as you practice you will be able to breathe this way for longer periods.

- Gently place your fingers in your ears and focus on the sound of the breath within your body.

- Have fun with this exercise! Imagine the soothing and rhythmic ocean within you, vast, powerful, and strong.

BIG ROUND TIRE BREATH

What Is Big Round Tire Breath and How Does It Help?

Big Round Tire Breath is an exercise that focuses on letting go and releasing. Because it slows down the breath, this exercise is calming to the mind and body. Have your kids try it for several rounds and notice how different they feel.

» *Also good for: relaxation and stress-busting*

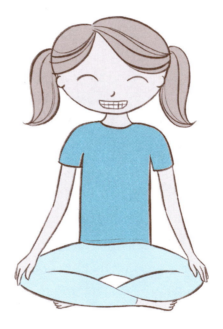

Slow and steady exhale

TIP: *Big Round Tire Breath can be practiced anywhere—such as when kids have to wait in a long line at the movies or at an amusement park.*

SIMPLE STEPS FOR KIDS

- Begin in a comfortable seated position: Sit comfortably in a chair, spine naturally erect, shoulders relaxed, hands resting on thighs, and feet flat on the floor.

- Take a deep breath in through your nose, filling up your entire torso—like a big round tire—with air.

- Pause and then slowly release the air through your teeth making a hissing sound, like a tire with a slow, steady leak.

- As you let the "air" slowly hiss out of your body, imagine any negative thoughts, fears, worries, or emotions leaving with it.

- Repeat for three to five rounds.

TACO TONGUE

What Is Taco Tongue?

While it certainly sounds silly, Taco Tongue is a breathing technique that has a cooling and calming effect on the body and nervous system. The long sides of the tongue are curled in to form a taco-like shape—hence the name, Taco Tongue.

How Does It Help?

Think of a puppy panting when he is playing; drawing cool air over his tongue is his way of cooling his body when it begins to warm from activity. When your kids practice Taco Tongue breathing, they create a straw- or tube-like shape with their tongue and draw air over its surface, cooling the tongue and the body. This sensation of cool air is invigorating, bringing the senses and, ultimately, the attention to the present moment, making this an excellent activity for developing focus and concentration.

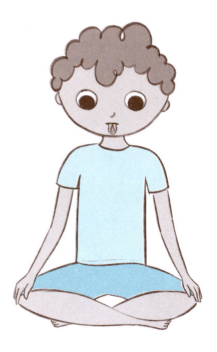

Taco Tongue also triggers a calming response in the nervous system. When the tongue is rolled into a straw-like shape, the intake of air (the breath) is immediately slowed down. Slowing the breath activates the parasympathetic nervous system, or "rest and digest" mode. (Essentially this statement is true of any of the breathing techniques where the breath is slowed down.) The result is a reduction in negative mind–body states such as anxiety or anger.

If your kids practice Taco Tongue several times daily, they'll be sharp, attentive, and cool as a cucumber (or should that be an avocado?).

» Also good for: focus and stress-busting

Roll the tongue

SIMPLE STEPS FOR KIDS

- Begin in a comfortable seated position, spine naturally erect. Relax your shoulders, arms, and face, and rest your hands in your lap.

- Curl both sides of the tongue inward, rolling it into a straw shape, like a taco.

- Slowly breathe in through the straw shape your tongue has formed.

- Once your inhale is complete, draw the tongue back into your mouth and relax it (allow it to unroll) as you exhale slowly through your nose.

- Repeat. As you practice Taco Tongue, gradually build to eight to twelve rounds per sitting.

TIP: *If your child is unable to curl her tongue lengthwise (many people are anatomically unable to do this), have her try the following:*

- Relax the jaw, allowing the mouth to drop open slightly.

- Rest the tip of the tongue behind the upper teeth.

- Inhale slowly through the space between the teeth.

- After completing the inhale, relax the tongue, close the mouth, and exhale through the nose. Repeat, building to eight to twelve rounds per sitting.

PART TWO

Hocus Pocus, I Can Focus

MEDITATION TECHNIQUES FOR CLEAR, BRIGHT, AND FOCUSED MINDS

D o you think you need magical powers to teach your kids how to meditate, or simply focus on one task at a time? Think again! This section of the book features fun and simple meditation tools designed to help kids direct their attention, from quick and easy methods to center and refocus inattentive kids, to longer meditation experiences that clear the mind and relax the body.

It can be hard for kids to focus today, with so many priorities and distractions—from sports to school to social media—competing for their attention. It's easy for kids to become frazzled and overwhelmed. This is where meditation can help! Often referred to as mindfulness, the practice of meditation is bringing one's complete attention to the present on a moment-to-moment basis. It's also a great tool to simply help kids center themselves and focus on important stuff like exams, homework, and lessons. For example, psychologists at the University of North Carolina[*] studying the effects of a meditation technique known as mindfulness found that meditation-trained participants showed a significant improvement in their critical cognitive skills and performed better in cognitive tests than a control group.

The benefits are not limited to the classroom. Athletic kids find meditation helpful too—honing the ability to stop and center oneself in the moment can be the difference between slugging the ball out of the ballpark or wildly swinging and striking out.

[*] University of North Carolina at Charlotte. "Brief meditative exercise helps cognition." ScienceDaily. www.sciencedaily.com/releases/2010/04/100414184220.htm (accessed November 27, 2017).

Will I Really Be Able to Get Them to Practice?

Most kids, when told that something is good for them, shy away from it. Not that they necessarily gravitate toward things that are bad for them, but "good" simply does not sound like "fun" to a kid. The activities featured in this chapter are designed to engage kids in a fun and playful way so they *enjoy* practicing meditation.

Remember

Many techniques in this book fall under more than one category. There are several helpful active meditation games in the Connect section (pages 161–177) that kids can play together—all of the kids I have taught are amazed (and proud) to learn they were meditating after playing. You may find a great approach in this section that doubles as a breath-awareness technique or chill-out tool. Explore the whole book and keep an open dialogue going with your kids about how each practice benefited them and how they might apply what they learned to different situations in their lives.

BALLOON BREATH

What Is Balloon Breath?

Balloon Breath is a breathing technique that slows down the breath while encouraging full and deep inhales and exhales to calm the mind and body.

How Does It Help?

Balloon Breath is great to use as a quick exercise to center and calm oneself during activities or to refocus before or during class. Linking physical movement to the breath encourages mind–body connection, a form of meditation or present-moment awareness resulting in improved concentration and self-regulation. The physical movement of raising the arms up overhead in this exercise allows more space in the torso to accommodate fuller and deeper breaths.

» *Also good for: breath control*

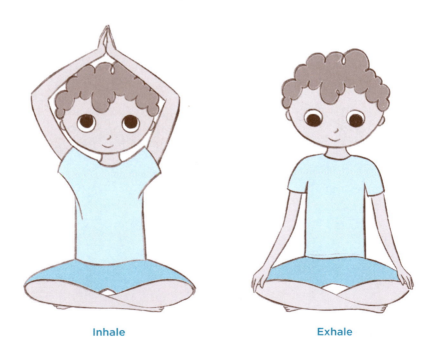

Inhale   Exhale

SIMPLE STEPS FOR KIDS

- Begin sitting comfortably, either on a chair or on the floor with the hands resting on the thighs. Relax the shoulders, arms, and face.

- Or, begin standing, feet hip-width distance apart, arms resting by the torso, shoulders and face relaxed.

- Begin to breathe in and out through the nose.

- Inhale, sweeping your arms up overhead. Imagine you are filling up a giant balloon.

- Exhale, slowly lowering your arms to rest in your lap or by your side.

- Repeat for several rounds.

- Get creative: Imagine the color of your balloon as you inflate it. Does thinking of a certain color make you feel more relaxed? Visualize releasing your balloon into the sky as you exhale. Where does your balloon go?

MELTING SNOWFLAKES

What Are Melting Snowflakes?

Does your child ever feel as if his mind is so full of thoughts, it is like a blustery snowstorm? Melting Snowflakes is a visualization technique that can help manage thoughts, clear the mind, and help one learn meditation. Treating each thought like a snowflake, one simply allows it to softly fall from the mind and melt away.

How Does It Help?

Meditation is quite simple, yet it can be overwhelming to learn. It's difficult to know just where to begin—particularly when the mind is full of thoughts swirling around. Fortunately, kids have the power to manage their thoughts and enjoy the clear-minded benefits that meditation offers. Melting Snowflakes is a wonderful tool that teaches how to chip away one thought, or snowflake, at a time—a much more manageable task than trying to clear the whole storm in one fell swoop.

» *Also good for: relaxation*

TIP: *If you notice your child is holding tension in her body, encourage her to relax by imagining the body as a giant snowflake gently melting in the sun. A relaxed mind and body go hand in hand, and, the more comfortable and relaxed the physical body, the easier it will be to focus on learning how to meditate and melt those pesky mental snowflakes away.*

SIMPLE STEPS FOR KIDS

- Begin in a comfortable position, either sitting or resting on your back.

- Close your eyes and take one to three breaths—breathing in through the nose and exhaling with an open-mouth sigh. Let go a little bit more with each exhale.

- Breathe normally and allow your attention to settle on your thoughts.

- As each thought arises, imagine it as a beautiful, delicate snowflake, gently falling from the sky.

- Visualize that snowflake falling to the ground and melting completely. Allow the thought to melt away along with this image of the snowflake melting.

- Repeat this visualization as each new thought arises. If several thoughts arise at once, simply choose one and follow the above steps to melt that thought away.

- Be patient with yourself. This technique may sound easy, but it can be challenging. Thoughts may storm at you initially, but with patience and practice, you will master them.

- Practice, practice, practice. The more you work on this technique, the easier it will become. You will enjoy longer gaps of peaceful meditation between those pesky thoughts.

- Each time a pesky thought does arise, know that it is normal. Simply reimagine it as a snowflake and allow it to melt away.

CENTERING

What Is Centering?

Centering is a technique that connects the mind and body, resulting in an immediate sense of calm and relaxation. Centering can be used to focus on an activity such as meditation, homework, or an important class or exam.

How Does It Help?

Centering stops the chatter of the mind, bringing us to the present moment. Eliminating distractions and promoting awareness, Centering empowers us to be calm, focused, and ready for anything.

» *Also good for: breath control*

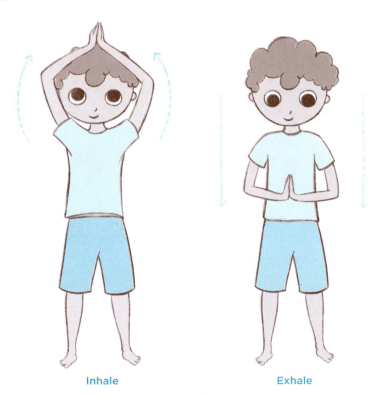

Inhale   Exhale

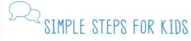

SIMPLE STEPS FOR KIDS

- Begin sitting comfortably on the floor or in a chair, or standing with the feet hip-width distance apart. Hold the spine naturally erect, and relax the arms, shoulders, and face.

- Inhale deeply as you sweep your arms out to the side and up overhead, bringing the palms to touch.

- Keep the palms pressed together and slowly slide them toward your heart as you exhale.

- Repeat for several rounds until you feel calm, relaxed, and centered.

TIP: *Each movement should last as long as each inhale or exhale. You can explain to your child like this: In this exercise, your breath acts like gas in a car; the car only moves if it's filled with fuel. Likewise, your body should only move when you are either inhaling or exhaling—no breath, no movement.*

SUNSHINE BREATH

What Is Sunshine Breath?

Sunshine Breath is an active breath exercise that links gentle body movements to your child's breath cycle.

How Does It Help?

By connecting movement to breath, kids learn about their breath cycle and can work toward slowing and controlling it. The physical movement in Sunshine Breath allows more space in the torso to encourage fuller and deeper breaths, calming the nervous system, body, and mind. Sunshine Breath can be used as a centering exercise and is excellent to practice before doing something that needs your child's full attention, such as meditation, a test, or a class.

» *Also good for: breath control*

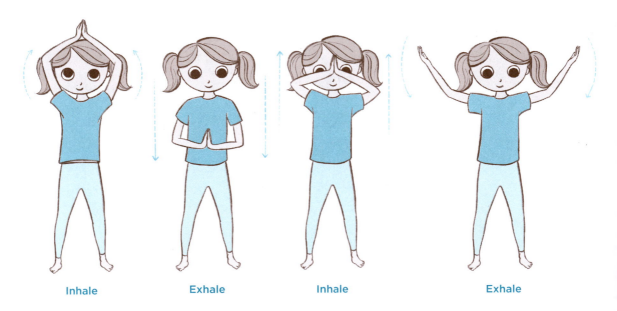

| Inhale | Exhale | Inhale | Exhale |

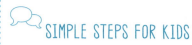 ## SIMPLE STEPS FOR KIDS

Sunshine Breath can be practiced standing or seated on the floor or in a chair.

STANDING: Stand up straight with both feet planted on the ground about hip-width distance apart. Slide the shoulder blades down your back and relax the arms by your torso.

FLOOR: Sit comfortably, either crisscross or kneeling. Hold the spine naturally erect, relax the shoulders, and rest your arms by your torso.

CHAIR: Sit comfortably with both feet planted on the floor, spine naturally erect. Relax the shoulders with the arms resting by the torso.

- Gently close your eyes, or softly gaze at a point in front of you.

- Turn your attention inward and begin to observe your natural breath as it flows in and out for a few rounds.

- On an inhale, sweep the arms up in a big circle until the palms meet high above your head.

- Exhale, keeping the palms pressed together and drawing them down toward the middle of your chest or heart.

- Inhale, keeping the palms pressed together and straightening the arms back up overhead.

- Exhale, circling the arms back down alongside the torso. This is one complete round. Repeat three to five full rounds.

- Sit quietly and enjoy the sensations created by this movement and deep breathing.

TIP: *Remind your child to link his body movement to his breath. Each movement should match his inhale and exhale. Like a car that does not move without gas, his body should not move without an in or out breath fueling it.*

TWISTER BREATH

What Is Twister Breath and How Does It Help?

Practicing Twister Breath helps balance the left and right hemispheres of the brain. It aids in slowing down the breath, calming the nervous system, and relieving stress, anxiety, and insomnia. Because it requires focus and coordination, this exercise is great for concentration.

» *Also good for: breath control*

TIPS:

- *Shoulders should be relaxed. If your child's arms become fatigued, she can use both hands and alternate blocking each nostril with the index finger of each hand.*

- *Simply using the index finger of each hand to close and release each nostril is recommended for younger children who have yet to develop the fine motor skills and coordination required to practice as outlined.*

- *If your child is left-handed, then reverse this exercise. Using the left hand, block off the left nostril with the thumb and then the right nostril with the ring and pinky fingers.*

SIMPLE STEPS FOR KIDS

- Begin in a comfortable upright position, either seated on the floor in crisscross position or kneeling, or in a chair. Keep your spine naturally erect but relaxed.

- Rest your left hand in your lap and raise your right hand toward your face. Rest your right index and middle fingers at the top of your nose, between the eyebrows, and gently close off your right nostril by lightly pressing the outside of it with your thumb.

- Inhale through your left nostril, and then close the left nostril by lightly pressing it with your ring and little fingers.

- Release your thumb from your right nostril and exhale slowly and fully through the right nostril.

- Keeping the right nostril open, inhale fully, and then close it off with the thumb.

- Release the ring and little fingers from your left nostril and exhale slowly and fully out of the left nostril. This completes one cycle. Repeat three to five times.

- Rest your hand in your lap and commence normal breathing. Sit with the eyes closed, enjoying the sensations of balance and serenity this exercise brings.

SNOW GLOBE MEDITATION

What Is Snow Globe Meditation?

Snow Globe Meditation is a fun craft project that teaches kids how to settle or quiet the mind when it is too busy or overwhelmed with a lot of thoughts and/or feelings.

How Does It Help?

Sometimes we have so many thoughts swirling around all at once that we cannot begin to think straight. This is not only overwhelming and exhausting but also unhealthy for the mind and the body. Meditation can help by giving the mind a rest, so to speak. Learning to meditate and introducing regular practice helps kids clear their minds and alleviate feelings of stress or anxiety.

» *Also good for: relaxation*

What Do You Need?

- A small glass jar with a lid (rinse an old jelly, infant food, or mason jar)
- Glitter (several colors if possible)
- Liquid glycerin

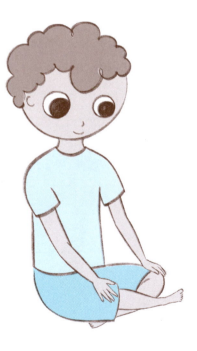
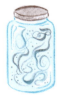

Thoughts settle with glitter

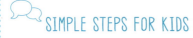

SIMPLE STEPS FOR KIDS

- Fill just over one-half of a clean glass jar with lukewarm tap water.

- Adding liquid glycerin, fill to about one-quarter inch from top.

- Tighten the lid on the jar and gently shake until the liquids mix together.

- The clear fluid in the jar is like your mind in its clear, natural state. Place the jar in front of you and remove the lid. Take a moment to focus on your mind. When a thought arises, place a pinch of glitter in the jar to represent that thought. You can use a different color glitter (if you have it) for each thought or type of thought you are having (for example, sad, angry, scared, and so forth). Once you feel ready, place the lid firmly back on the jar and give it a shake. Watch all of your "thoughts" swirl around in the jar . . . isn't that just how your mind feels sometimes?

- Settle the jar on a flat surface in front of you and sit comfortably and quietly. Begin to breathe slowly as you watch the glitter settle toward the bottom of the jar. As the glitter slows down and settles, allow your thoughts to do the same.

TIP: *Keep your child's jar and let him use it whenever he feels overwhelmed by thoughts, or when he simply needs to clear his mind and relax.*

DROPPING IN

What Is Dropping In?

Dropping In is an effective exercise to quickly gain focus, or "drop in" to the present moment. It is also a helpful tool that encourages longer meditations or active meditation sessions (meaning kids can do it when they are physically active, walking, and so forth). This exercise is especially helpful for kids who may have trouble concentrating in traditional seated meditation.

How Does It Help?

Present-moment awareness has been known to calm the mind and quiet ruminative, obsessive, or negative thought patterns, reducing feelings of distress and encouraging a positive mood. Dropping In is highly effective as a quick fix to refocus your child's attention on the present moment when she finds her mind wandering.

» *Also good for: relaxation*

TIP: *In the beginning, it will be natural for your child's mind to create stories about the sensations she observes. For example, she might hear a neighbor's music playing and create a story such as "Wow, she is playing her music really loudly today. I hope she turns it down when I am doing my homework later so I can concentrate. I don't even like this song—why she listens to this I have no idea. I used to like this artist, but I like so and so now . . ." This is what the mind does all day long, without our being aware of it. One sound, one smell, one experience can trigger an entire monologue inside our minds that can go on for minutes or even hours! The Dropping In technique retrains the mind to stay in the present moment by focusing on sensations as they are and not thinking about them. In this example, encourage your child to simply notice the music's sounds and vibrations, without wondering about where it is coming from or who is singing.*

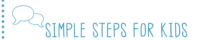

SIMPLE STEPS FOR KIDS

SEATED OR RECLINED

- Begin in a comfortable seated position, on the floor or in a chair, or lying comfortably on your back. Use cushions and/or blankets as needed to be as comfortable as possible.

- Gently close your eyes and take a few slow, deep breaths.

- As you begin to relax, notice any sensations you are experiencing, such as where your body is making contact with the chair or floor, or the sensation of the air on your skin. Can you feel the sun or a breeze from an air conditioner? Are there any sounds? Listen for obvious ones—and then listen deeper for sounds beyond the area where you are practicing. Observe and examine each sensation fully before moving on to the next.

WALKING

This technique can be practiced anywhere—walking to school, strolling around the mall, hiking through a park or nature trail, and so on.

- Center yourself by taking a few deep breaths in and out.

- Begin to walk slowly and mindfully. Notice each step you take. Observe in detail as each part of your foot makes contact with the ground. Notice the pressure and sensation of each and every step you take.

- Take in your surroundings. Notice in every detail—the color of the sky, cloud formations, and the different shades of green in each leaf.

- What other sensations can you observe? The air touching your skin? The sounds around you? Be open to different sensations and present with each one as it occurs, approaching each with curiosity as though observing it for the first time.

Guiding Your Child through Dropping In

The first time your child tries this meditation, she may be unsure what to focus on or need some direction. To guide your child through this exercise and help her isolate the many sensations around her, try reading the following helpful cues to your child:

PHYSICAL

- Feel any objects with which your body makes contact: the floor, a chair, another body part, and so on. Notice differences between each side of your body—how each feels, pressure at contact points, temperature, and any clothing touching your skin.
- Focus on where the skin makes contact with the air around you. What is the temperature? Is there a wind or breeze? Any other sensations?

AUDITORY

- Listen to the sounds around you, from a buzzing mosquito to a neighbor's music. Don't attach a story to what you hear; simply observe the sounds.

OLFACTORY

- Notice any smells around you.

- How do these odors make your nose feel? Notice your nostrils flaring, mouth watering, and so forth. Whatever your physical response is to the smell, don't create a story about it. Stay present and observe every detail of each sensation.

VISUAL

- Observe the details of your surroundings, such as the color of the sky and the changing shapes of the clouds.

BREATH

- Focus on your breath. Be aware of the depth of the breath, which body parts move with each inhale and exhale, how they move, the temperature of the air, and the sensations created as the breath enters and leaves your body.

SPIDERWEB BREATH

What Is Spiderweb Breath?

Spiderweb Breath is a visualization technique that encourages deep breathing while offering a strong meditation component to calm and relax the body and mind.

How Does It Help?

This activity helps kids connect with and observe their breath. Sometimes observing the breath alone can become boring; adding the visual element of a spiderweb can make it easier for kids to stay present with the breath and enjoy the many benefits meditation offers.

» *Also good for: breath control and relaxation*

TIP: *Be creative: Kids do not have to visualize a spiderweb if they don't want to! They can imagine a beam of light or a favorite color washing through them. The important thing is to follow the breath on its complete journey using the space between their eyebrows and their belly button as a guiding point to help them breathe slowly and fully.*

SIMPLE STEPS FOR KIDS

- Begin in a comfortable position, either seated or lying down.

- Gently close your eyes and begin to reflect inwardly.

- Breathe naturally, in and out through your nose.

- Slowly begin to deepen your breath by gradually increasing the length of each inhale and exhale.

- Continue breathing slowly and deeply as you shift your attention to the space between your eyebrows. The next time you breathe in, imagine that the breath is a shiny silver spiderweb, entering your body at the point between your eyebrows.

- Follow the spiderweb as it flows through your body all the way to your belly button.

- As you breathe out, imagine the shiny silver spiderweb gently pulling your belly button in toward your spine, flowing back up through your body, and out the space between your eyebrows.

- Continue to breathe this way for five minutes. Build the length of time you practice each day until you can practice for thirty to sixty minutes.

TAKE TEN

What Is Take Ten?

Take Ten is a breathing technique that invites relaxation and sharpens the ability to focus.

How Does It Help?

Take Ten is helpful if kids have a lot of mental chatter happening and need to shift their focus. Benefits of practicing Take Ten include stress reduction and increased mental clarity. Take Ten can be practiced lying down if your child is having trouble falling asleep. Who says you need to count sheep? Count your breath instead!

» *Also good for: breath control, stress-busting, and relaxation*

SIMPLE STEPS FOR KIDS

- Begin in a comfortable seated position, either in a chair with both feet on the floor, or in crisscross position (use yoga blocks or blankets under your hips and/or knees if your hips are tight). Be sure the spine is straight and the shoulders, arms, and face are relaxed.

- Gently close your eyes.

- Observe the breath. Do not try to control it; just let the in and out breaths occur naturally.

- Begin to count each breath, counting off each complete round by saying to yourself, "I am breathing in, one," "I am breathing out, one," "I am breathing in, two," "I am breathing out, two," and so on.

- Continue to do this until you complete ten rounds of breaths. After you reach ten, return to one and count out ten full rounds once again.

- This is not as easy as it sounds! Your mind will wander off and begin thinking about things. This is perfectly natural. When you notice this occurring, congratulate yourself for catching the deviation and begin counting the breath once again. *But there's a catch:* You will need to begin at one again!

- Have fun with this activity and try it often. See how far you can go before your mind tunes out.

- Can you make it to ten breaths without a mental diversion? Great! Challenge yourself by increasing the number.

FOCUSED BREATHING

What Is Focused Breathing?

Focused Breathing is a relaxation technique that uses the breath as a focal point.

How Does It Help?

Observing the breath provides an anchor to the present moment. Each inhale and exhale links one moment to the next. When kids concentrate on their breath, their mind focuses on the present moment, clearing away unrelated distractions or thoughts. A clear mind allows kids to be fully present and to zero in on important stuff such as homework, sports, and hobbies.

» *Also good for: breath control, stress-busting, and relaxation*

 SIMPLE STEPS FOR KIDS

- Begin in a comfortable seated position. Be sure your spine is straight and your shoulders, arms, and legs are relaxed.

- Close your eyes and perform a quick Body Scan (page 138) to be sure you are comfortable and relaxed. If you feel tension anywhere, do what you can to relax that area. This may be as simple as consciously relaxing a muscle, changing your position or where you are sitting, or using a prop such as a pillow or blanket.

- Once you feel comfortable, close your eyes and focus on the natural rhythm of your breath. Do not force it or try to control it; simply observe how you breathe naturally.

- Keeping your eyes gently closed, begin to follow the breath's journey in great detail.

- Notice the area around the nostrils as the breath enters your body—temperature, sensation, and so on.

- Follow your breath through the nasal passages, to the back of the throat, and down into the lungs.

- Notice your collarbones expanding.

- Follow your breath as it expands the lungs. Notice the ribs expanding too. Do they expand at the sides as well as the front and back of the torso?

- Follow the breath as you exhale, noticing the lungs relaxing as the air expels. Observe the ribs and collarbones relaxing too.

- Notice any sensations as the air exits the nostrils.

- Keep observing each step of each breath for three to five minutes. Be as detailed as you can.

- If your mind wanders off, simply redirect the focus to the sensations and passage of your breath and begin again.

- You may wish to add visual elements to this breathing exercise. Visualize tension or anxiety leaving the body as you exhale. Breathe in calmness and relaxation as you inhale.

- Visualize a color representing vitality as you breathe in, and another color representing relaxation as you breathe out.

- If you prefer a verbal association, simply think of the words *calm* and *relax* as you breathe in and out.

MANTRA

What Is a Mantra and How Does It Help?

Meditation is a helpful tool that can calm and soothe the body, mind, and nervous system. It also relieves symptoms of stress or anxiety and improves kids' ability to focus. But meditating can be hard! Using a mantra—a word or phrase usually linked to the in and out breath—can help kids master and enjoy the many benefits of meditation. Think of a Mantra as an anchor that keeps its ship (your child) firmly anchored in the present moment, rather than drifting aimlessly in an ocean of thought.

» *Also good for: breath control, stress-busting, and relaxation*

Mantra Box

Is your child having trouble coming up with a Mantra that inspires? Here are some suggestions:

"I am breathing in . . . I am breathing out"

"I am breathing in energy . . . I am breathing out and relaxing"

"I am breathing in the color yellow . . . I am breathing out the color green"

"I am breathing in radiant sunshine . . . I am breathing out radiant sunshine"

"Breathing in, my body expands . . . Breathing out, my body relaxes"

"Breathing in, my body feels light . . . Breathing out, my body feels lighter"

"Breathing in, I feel calm . . . Breathing out, I feel relaxed"

SIMPLE STEPS FOR KIDS

- Choose a mantra that works for you, one that you believe and can easily visualize. (See Mantra Box, at left, for ideas.)

- Begin in a comfortable seated position in a chair or on the floor. If you're sitting on the floor, prop yourself up on a pillow or bolster to ensure you can sit comfortably for longer periods.

- Gently close the eyes and turn your attention inward.

- Observe your breath as it flows in and out of your body.

- When you feel ready to begin, say your mantra in your head as you breathe in.

- As you breathe out, repeat your mantra in your head.

- If your mind wanders off and you catch yourself thinking about something other than your mantra, simply let go of the thoughts and refocus your attention on your breath. Observe your breath for a few rounds and then begin repeating your mantra again.

TIPS:

- *A mantra does not have to be an entire phrase, nor does it need to be a different word for each inhale and exhale. It can be a single word that your child repeats with each in and out breath, such as* **happy, strength, smile, calm, relax, serenity,** *or* **sunshine.**

- *Encourage your child to focus on positives rather than negatives. For example, if he is feeling blue or sad and uses a mantra such as, "I am breathing in happiness," he should follow it with a positive statement such as, "I am breathing out and* **letting go**," *rather than, "I am breathing out sadness."*

PART THREE

Stress Busters and Energy Equalizers

ALL ABOUT:
ACTIVITIES TO RELEASE STRESS AND REGULATE ENERGY LEVELS

Explode like a firework, shake like a milkshake, or roar like a lion! All of the techniques in this section teach kids how to regulate stress and have more control over their body and energy levels. Many adults view stress as a grown-up problem and have trouble imagining that children are as busy and stressed out as they are! The pressures of homework, test performance, social anxieties, and even athletic competition result in unwanted tension negatively impacting kids' minds, bodies, and spirits. The exercises in this section help kids release built-up stress and regulate their energy levels to bring them to a happier and more mindful place.

Techniques designed to release stress are also an ideal outlet for pent-up energy. Many children simply don't know what to "do" with their bodies, resulting in inattentive, impulsive, restless, or fidgety behavior. Connecting the mind and body via fluid movement, the activities here encourage kids to gently stretch, move, and flex the physical body with awareness and control, resulting in reflective behavior and the awareness to recognize and manage reflexive patterns. And, on the other end of the energy spectrum, active and playful techniques are energizing and provide the perfect remedy for kids bogged down by a midafternoon slump.

In a classroom environment the following activities provide kids the opportunity to release pent-up stress and/or excess energy, re-center, and refocus, preparing them to learn and be more productive. At home and at play, children develop the ability to manage stress and regulate energy levels on their own.

LION'S BREATH

What Is Lion's Breath and How Does It Help?

Lion's Breath is a fantastic exercise to release tension and stress. It stretches the mouth, jaw, tongue, eyes, and hands—all common areas where tension can be found. Practicing Lion's Breath is also a lot of fun!

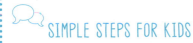 SIMPLE STEPS FOR KIDS

- Begin by kneeling on the floor or sitting upright, spine naturally erect. If sitting on the knees is too uncomfortable for your joints, then sitting in a chair is fine—be sure to sit nice and straight with both feet planted on the floor. Hands should be relaxed, resting comfortably in the lap.

- Inhale deeply through your nose.

- Open your mouth wide, stick out your tongue, and exhale strongly while making a "ha" sound.

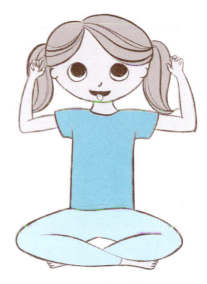

Roar! Make noise!

- Turn your eyes to look up toward the ceiling and stretch your hands and fingers to frame either side of your face like a lion's bushy mane.

- Repeat two or three times.

- Notice how you feel after practicing Lion's Breath.

BUMBLEBEE BREATH

What Is Bumblebee Breath?

Bumblebee Breath is a fun breathing technique where kids make the sound of a bumblebee. Tickling the mouth and lips, Bumblebee Breath fills the whole body with the vibration and energy of kids' own breaths.

How Does It Help?

Bumblebee Breath helps shift the attention inward by shutting off outside distractions and focusing on the vibration of the breath. A soothing practice, it results in feelings of relaxation and calm. Bumblebee Breath is also empowering, reminding kids of the control and energy they already have inside of them.

» *Also good for: breath control*

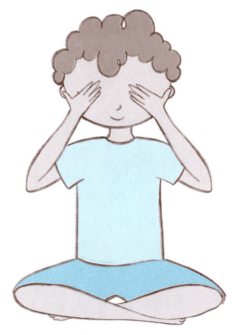

Buzz like a bee!

SIMPLE STEPS FOR KIDS

- Begin in a comfortable seated position, either on the floor or in a chair. Sit up nice and tall, yet relaxed.

- Cover your ears with your thumbs, blocking any outside sounds. Gently wrap the remaining four fingers over your closed eyes; this will help you really focus on what is happening inside of you.

- Take a big breath in, filling up with air until the belly expands. Exhale through the nose, keeping your lips closed, making a humming sound for the duration of your exhale.

- Keeping your eyes closed, return to normal breathing and gently rest your hands in your lap. Observe the sensations the sound has created in your body.

- Repeat for several rounds, gradually building to five to ten rounds per sitting.

- If you feel dizzy or light-headed while practicing Bumblebee Breath (or any breathing exercise), take a break and resume normal breathing.

- Reflect on the experience. What did you feel when you practiced Bumblebee Breath? Did you feel the buzzing sensation or vibration anywhere else, or only on your lips? How about your tongue? What happened when the breath and sound finished? Could you still feel the vibration? How did it make you feel after? Did your mind or thoughts wander while you were practicing?

WATERWHEEL

What Is Waterwheel?

Waterwheel is an active breathing exercise that engages the physical body in a pump-like action.

How Does It Help?

Similar to the action the diaphragm makes when breathing, the physical movement the body makes practicing Waterwheel encourages full diaphragmatic breathing. Waterwheel actively engages the abdominal muscles, so kids get a little bit of a core workout too—a strong core supports the lower back and helps maintain good posture, which allows one to breathe better. The physical pumping action of the legs in this exercise encourages kids to take deeper and fuller breaths.

» *Also good for: breath control*

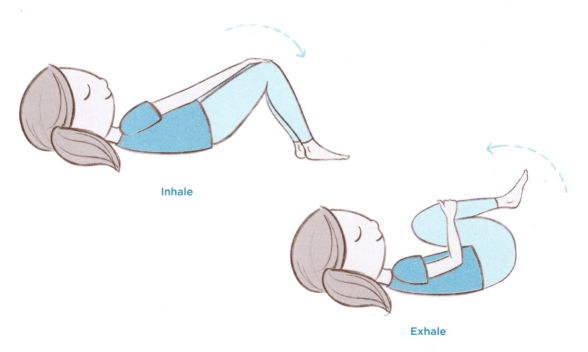

Inhale

Exhale

SIMPLE STEPS FOR KIDS

- Begin by lying on your back.

- Hug your knees to your chest and press your lower back to the floor. Keep both hips in contact with the floor the entire time you practice Waterwheel.

- Slide your hands to the tops of the knees and, as you inhale, drop your feet toward the floor, just below the hips.

- Exhale and hug the knees back into the chest, squeezing all of the air out of your lungs as you bring in the knees.

- Inhale and slowly lower the feet back to the floor.

- Exhale and draw the knees back in toward the chest.

- Repeat for several rounds. Your movements should be rhythmic and smooth, like a waterwheel pumping in sync with your breath.

ELEPHANT SHOWER

What Is Elephant Shower and How Does It Help?

Elephant Shower is an active breathing posture that has two components: a stretching one to energize the body, and a releasing one to encourage relaxation and letting go. The releasing part of Elephant Shower is actually a type of physical inversion, meaning the head is lower than the heart, which is known to be rejuvenating. Elephant Shower is great to use when kids feel fidgety and have a lot of excess energy. It is a positive way to release some of that energy, become centered, stretch, relax, and feel good.

» *Also good for: breath control*

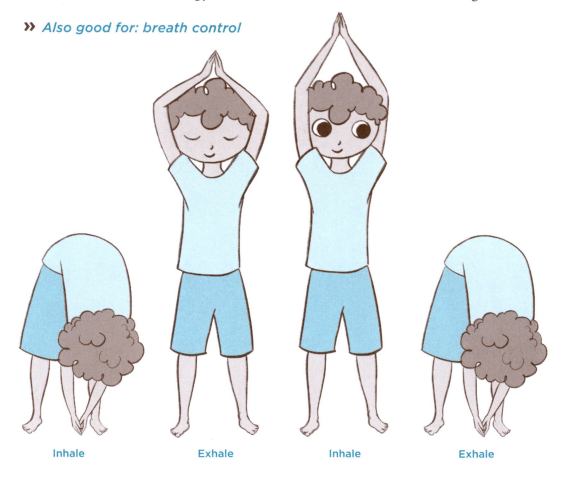

Inhale   Exhale   Inhale   Exhale

SIMPLE STEPS FOR KIDS

- Begin standing with your feet slightly wider than hip-width distance apart.

- Clasp your hands together to make an elephant trunk with your arms.

- Fold at your hips and allow your head and arms to hang heavy.

- Pretend you have a huge watering hole at your feet and make slurping sounds as you drink some water up through your trunk.

- When you have had enough to drink, take a *big* breath in as you take one final slurp through your trunk.

- As you exhale, stand up tall, lifting your trunk high up in the air over your head—spraying the water from your trunk like a shower.

- Take a big breath in, stretching your trunk high over your head.

- As you breathe out, lower your trunk, folding your body over your legs, allowing your arms and head to hang heavy once more.

- Repeat for three rounds.

- Get creative. Imagine your elephant is spraying something other than water, such as your favorite color, happiness, glitter, or giggles! You can shower yourself with anything you like.

- Have fun! Shower your friends with happiness, glitter, and giggles too.

HORSE BREATH

What Is Horse Breath?

Horse Breath is a breathing technique also known as pursed-lip breathing. While it is a lot of fun to do, this exercise is more than mere horseplay and boasts plenty of health benefits.

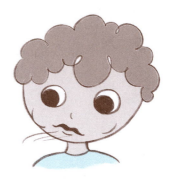

How Does It Help?

Horse Breath is an excellent exercise to regulate kids' breathing if they find themselves short of breath. Engagement of the

Lips flop on exhale

abdominal muscles during the exhale causes a deeper exhale to occur, automatically followed by a deeper inhale—regulating and slowing down the breath. Horse Breath also relaxes the mouth and jaw area, places we commonly carry tension without being aware of it!

SIMPLE STEPS FOR KIDS

- Begin in a comfortable seated position.

- Inhale normally through the nose.

- Keep the lips relaxed and in a rested position (loosely closed), and exhale through the mouth. The lips should vibrate and flutter as the air passes through them, sounding a little like a horse when he flutters his lips.

- Inhaling through the nose, repeat for a few rounds, building to three to five rounds per session.

- Observe the rest of your body when you breathe this way. Do you feel your abdominals engage as you exhale? Do you naturally breathe a little deeper after practicing for a few rounds?

FUNNY BUNNY BREATH

What Is Funny Bunny Breath?

Funny Bunny Breath is an energizing breath exercise.

How Does It Help?

Funny Bunny Breath serves as a quick pick-me-up when kids feel a little sluggish. The quick intake of oxygen revives the mind and body; however, kids should take care not to overdo it. They should *never* complete more than three to five rounds of Funny Bunny Breath at a time, and should slowly build to this amount, beginning with just one round.

» *Also good for: focus*

SIMPLE STEPS FOR KIDS

- Begin by sitting on your knees; if kneeling is uncomfortable or difficult, then sit crisscross on the floor or upright in a chair.

- Rest your hands on your thighs.

- Exhale fully through the mouth making an "ah" sound until all the air is out.

- Close your mouth, wrinkle your nose like a bunny sniffing a carrot, and take three quick inhalations through the nose.

- Open the mouth and exhale fully with an "ah" sound.

- As you gain experience and become comfortable with this breathing technique, build to three to five rounds of Funny Bunny Breath per session as needed. Remember to *slowly* build to a higher number of rounds when practicing any breathing technique.

FIREWORK BREATH

What Is Firework Breath?

Firework Breath is a fun, active breathing exercise that is great for shaking off excess energy or silliness.

How Does It Help?

Sometimes kids have a lot of excess energy buzzing around inside of them, making it hard to focus or concentrate on important things, such as schoolwork. Firework Breath uses the body and the breath to harness and release some of that energy, making it easy for kids to sit, focus, do great work, and learn.

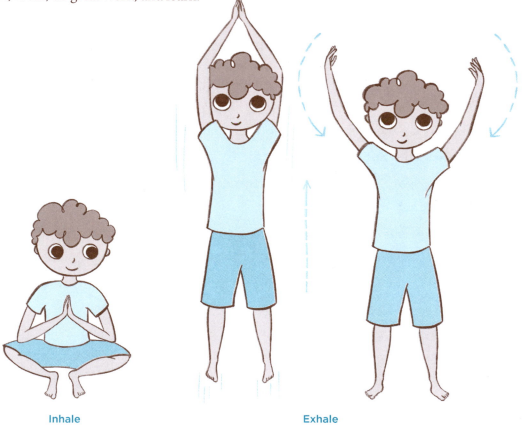

Inhale   Exhale

SIMPLE STEPS FOR KIDS

- Bending the knees, lower into a squat position.

- Draw your hands to your heart center with the palms pressed together. This is the tip of your firework launcher.

- Take a deep breath in through the nose, filling up your lungs.

- Launch your firework! Keep your palms pressed together as you shoot your arms straight up like a missile and jump to a standing position. Then spread the arms and legs out wide, like an exploding firework. Breathe out loudly through an open mouth as your firework explodes: "Pah!"

- Imagine what color and type of firework you are. Imagine how bright and dynamic you are.

LOCOMOTIVE

What Is Locomotive?

Locomotive is a nice, active breathing exercise that also gently stretches and flexes the spine. Linking movement to the breath and making the sounds of a train, Locomotive is also a present-moment awareness exercise.

How Does It Help?

Gently flexing and stretching the spine allows for better movement, mobility, and posture. Having good posture is healthy for our skeletal and muscular systems and creates space in our torsos so we can breathe fully and deeply. Practicing Locomotive also has meditative benefits: Matching the movement to the breath connects the mind and the body, while the "chhh" sound made while exhaling is great for releasing tension from the body.

>> *Also good for: focus*

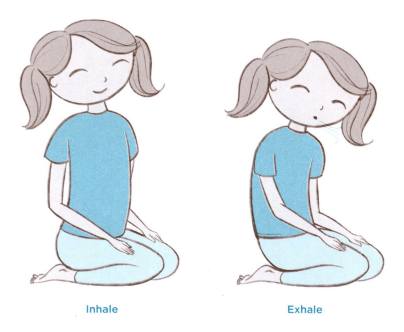

Inhale   Exhale

SIMPLE STEPS FOR KIDS

- Begin in a comfortable seated position, either sitting on the knees or crisscross on the floor, or seated on a chair.

- Rest your hands, palms down, on your thighs or knees.

- As you inhale through your nose, push your chest and belly forward as your butt and shoulders curl back, making a C shape with your spine.

- Exhale through your lips, making a "chhh" sound, as you pull your belly button in toward your spine, tuck in your tailbone and chin, and curl your spine into a C shape in the opposite direction.

- Repeat for several rounds.

- Play around with making your train travel at different speeds and notice how it makes you feel.

THUNDERSTORM

What Is Thunderstorm and How Does It Help?

Thunderstorm is a fun way to work all of the tension out of your child's body, preparing her for relaxation. It is also a great way to harness and release any extra energy your child may have, preparing her to settle in and focus on something important, such as a class or test.

 SIMPLE STEPS FOR KIDS

- Begin sitting on your knees and lightly tap on your legs, torso, shoulders, and head with your fingertips. The rain is beginning to lightly fall.

- Increase the tapping as the rain becomes harder.

- Lightly pat the floor with your palms as the rain becomes even harder. (Alternating the palms will create the sound of rain.)

- Pat your thighs to create the sound of even stronger rainfall.

- Pound your palms on the floor to make thunder. (Pounding both palms at the same time will simulate thunder.)

- Sit up and skim the palms together in an up-and-down motion to make lightning.

- Switch between rain, thunder, and lightning.

- Begin to slow the rain back down to a sprinkle, making the raindrops get lighter and lighter with each moment.

- Stretch out on the floor like a big, giant puddle left over from the storm and rest for up to five minutes.

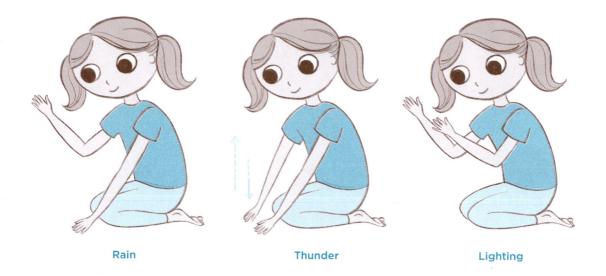

Rain   Thunder   Lighting

TIP: *For additional fun variations on this relaxation technique for kids, see the exercises Milkshake (page 104) and Spaghetti Boil (page 106).*

MILKSHAKE

What Is Milkshake and How Does It Help?

Milkshake is a fun way to shake away stress and help your body feel loose, limber, and *great!*

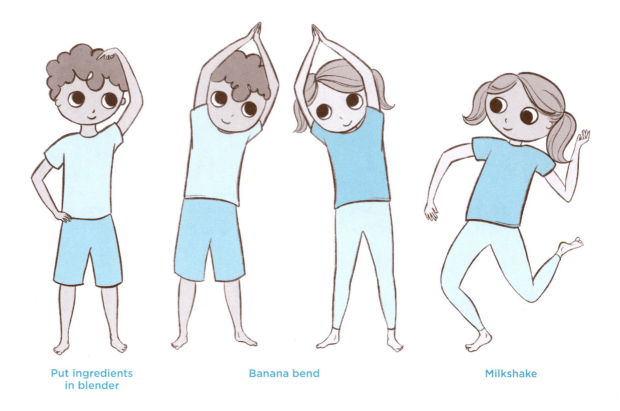

Put ingredients
in blender

Banana bend

Milkshake

TIP: *For similar exercises, try Thunderstorm (page 102) and Spaghetti Boil (page 106).*

SIMPLE STEPS FOR KIDS

- First, imagine what ingredients you would like in your milkshake. You can put anything you like in it—for example, bananas, yogurt, and milk.

- Imagine the top of the blender is the top of your head. Reach up and pour the milk inside your blender.

- Now add the yogurt.

- Stretch both hands overhead and lean to the right making a banana shape. Come back to the center and stretch up tall before leaning to the left like a banana. When you return to the center, place the banana inside your blender.

- Gently pat the top of your head to be sure the lid is on.

- Turn on the blender and shake your milkshake! Shake your legs and arms, wiggle your shoulders, and run in place. Shake-shake-shake your ingredients as fast as you can.

- Begin to reduce your blender's speed, your movements becoming slower and slower.

- Lower your yummy liquid milkshake onto the floor like a giant puddle.

- Stretch your body, reaching your arms up overhead, and point your toes—making a long straw out of your body for drinking the milkshake.

- Finally, relax your entire body, resting your hands on your belly, full and happy after enjoying your delicious milkshake.

- Rest here for up to five minutes.

SPAGHETTI BOIL

What Is Spaghetti Boil and How Does It Help?

Spaghetti Boil is a fun way to shake all the tension out of your child's body, preparing him for relaxation. It is also a positive way to harness and release any extra energy, anxieties, or silliness your child may have, preparing him to settle in and focus on the things in front of him.

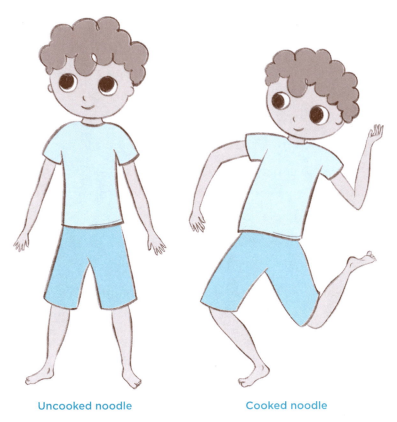

Uncooked noodle   Cooked noodle

TIP: *Teachers can perform a cooked noodle test! Shake each child's arms to test how floppy and well cooked her noodle is. Try Thunderstorm (page 102) and Milkshake (page 104) for variations of this technique.*

SIMPLE STEPS FOR KIDS

- Begin standing up tall, arms relaxed by your side. Now stiffen yourself from fingertips to toes, like a hard uncooked spaghetti noodle.

- Maintaining this stiffness, slowly begin to walk in a circle around a "pot" of water—arms and legs straight like a robot—your spaghetti noodle is still hard!

- Imagine the water in the pot getting warmer as it begins to boil. As the water gets warmer, your spaghetti noodle gets softer.

- As the water builds to a boil, move a little faster in the circle.

- Once the water is boiling, your noodle should be soft, floppy, and swirling around the pot. Loosen and relax your body, and move faster and faster in your circle.

- Now imagine the pot has been turned off and the boiling slows to a simmer. Slow down your body but stay floppy like a cooked noodle.

- Slowly lower your cooked noodle onto the floor and lie there all floppy.

- Rest for up to five minutes, allowing your noodle to cool down.

SUN BREATH

What Is Sun Breath?

Sun Breath is an energizing breath exercise.

How Does It Help?

Energizing breath exercises such as Sun Breath can wake kids up and give them a little energy when they're feeling groggy. They can also be a fun way to release any tension or excess energy kids may have. Sun Breath is especially good for releasing tension in the jaw and mouth area—common places people carry tension without being aware of it!

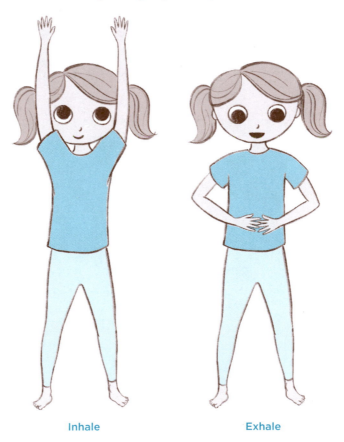

Inhale   Exhale

SIMPLE STEPS FOR KIDS

- Begin standing comfortably with the feet about hip-width distance apart.

- Inhale through your nose as you reach your hands toward the sky, as if you were going to grab hold of the sun with both hands.

- Quickly pull your hands back toward you, palms flat and facing the middle of your torso as you open your mouth and exhale, making a "ha!" sound. Imagine you are pulling the energy and power of the sun into your own core, or power center.

- Practice for a few rounds.

- Observe how you feel. Do you feel more energized? Do you feel bright and happy like the sun?

FUEL YOUR MOVES

What Is Fuel Your Moves?

Fuel Your Moves is an exercise where kids do exactly that—fuel their moves by connecting each movement to either an in or an out breath.

How Does It Help?

Connecting movement to breath does two things: It slows down the breath, resulting in feelings of relaxation, and it links the mind to the physical body, a form of meditation and present-moment awareness that promotes calmness and an ability to focus. The gentle physical movements in Fuel Your Moves are great tension relievers and provide a mini-break for the mind and body after using a computer or sitting for long periods of time.

» *Also good for: breath control and focus*

 SIMPLE STEPS FOR KIDS

- Begin sitting comfortably on the floor or in a chair, or standing, feet hip-width distance apart. Your spine should be naturally erect, and your arms and shoulders relaxed.

- Linking each of your inhales and exhales to a movement, follow the guide on the following pages, repeating each move for a total of three to five full rounds before moving on to the next.

- Remember: Each movement should last for the duration of each inhale or exhale. Just like gas fuels a car, your breath is what fuels your body to move in this exercise—no breath, no movement!

SHOULDER SHRUGS

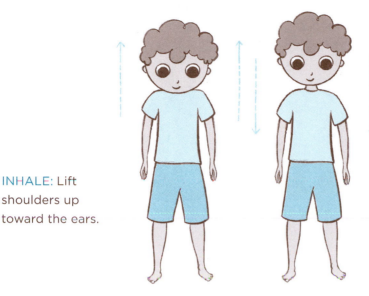

INHALE: Lift shoulders up toward the ears.

EXHALE: Lower shoulders, sliding the blades down the back.

SHOULDER ROLLS

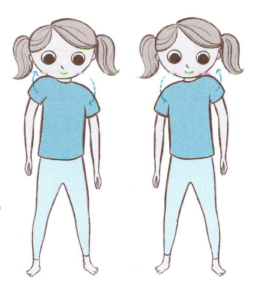

INHALE: Roll your right shoulder forward and up toward your ear. At the same time, drop your left shoulder back and down.

EXHALE: Roll your left shoulder forward and up toward your ear. At the same time, drop your right shoulder back and down.*

* Switch directions when repeating this exercise.

CHIN DROP

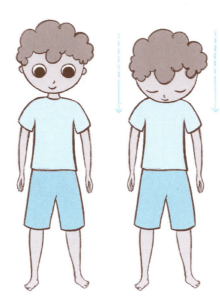

INHALE: Look straight ahead, keeping the chin level with the floor.

EXHALE: Drop your chin toward your chest, stretching the back of the neck.

NECK ROLLS

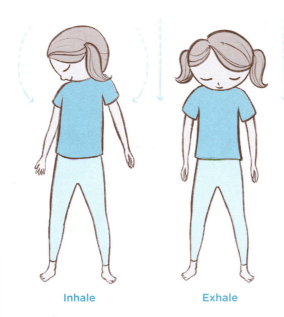

Inhale

Exhale

INHALE: Look straight ahead, keeping chin level with the floor.

EXHALE: Drop chin to chest.

INHALE: Keeping the chin close to the chest, roll the chin toward the right shoulder.

EXHALE: Keeping the chin close to the chest, roll the chin back to center.

INHALE: Keeping the chin close to the chest, roll the chin to the left shoulder.

EXHALE: Keeping the chin close to the chest, roll the chin to the center of the chest and inhale as you float the head up to a neutral position, chin level with the floor.

GENTLE TWISTS

INHALE: Sweep the arms up overhead.

EXHALE: Lowering the arms, gently twist to the left. Keep your hips facing front as you twist the torso, shoulders, and head to the left.

INHALE: Return to center, sweeping the arms back overhead.

EXHALE: Lowering the arms, gently twist to the right. Keep your hips facing front as you twist the torso, shoulders, and head to the right.

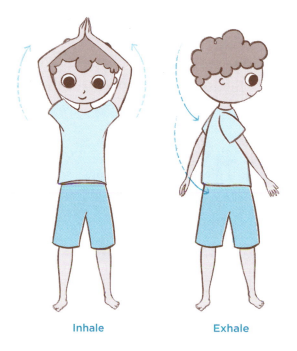

Inhale   Exhale

DRAGON BREATH

What Is Dragon Breath?

Has your child ever wished he could be a fire-breathing dragon? Well, he can! Dragon Breath is a fun way to relax the entire body and mind very quickly.

How Does It Help?

Dragon Breath is a great tool if your child is feeling stressed, or if he has been working hard physically or mentally and needs a break. The releasing, or letting go, element of Dragon Breath will have your child's mind and body feeling calm and relaxed in no time.

» *Also good for: breath control and relaxation*

TIP: *This is not like Lion's Breath (page 89), where your child roars and makes a lot of noise forcing the air out. To practice Dragon Breath, open the mouth and let the air flow out softly, like a fire-breathing dragon toasting a soft marshmallow. If the dragon forces out the air, he will burn the marshmallow to a crisp; if he breathes carefully and gently, the heat from his breath will toast the delicate marshmallow to perfection.*

SIMPLE STEPS FOR KIDS

- Begin in a comfortable position, either seated or lying on the floor.

- Alternatively, you can begin in child's pose: knees bent on the floor, torso resting on top of the thighs, and forehead resting on the floor. Allow the arms to lie on the floor alongside the torso, palms facing up.

- Take a deep breath in through the nose, filling the lungs until your belly pushes out.

- Open the mouth and let the air escape with an "aaaaaah."

- Repeat three to five times.

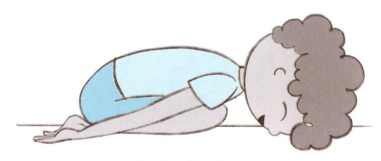

Fire-breathing dragon

BLOW IT AWAY

What Is Blow It Away?

Blow It Away is a creative visualization exercise that uses the breath to encourage letting go.

How Does It Help?

Blow It Away guides kids toward any negative feelings or thought patterns they may be harboring and gives them the opportunity to peacefully let them go. Using the exhale, which is the body letting go of stuff it no longer needs (carbon dioxide), they can also let go of nonphysical stuff, such as worries and anxieties.

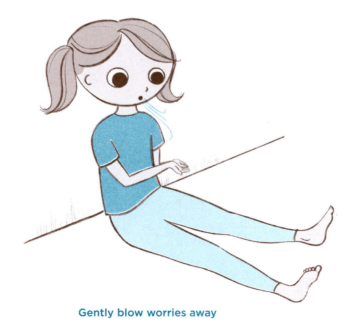

Gently blow worries away

TIP: *Teachers: Use different colored feathers to represent thoughts, feelings, or worries. Place these in kids' cupped hands and ask them to gently "blow away" each one.*

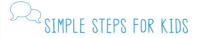

SIMPLE STEPS FOR KIDS

- Begin in a comfortable seated position.

- Cup your hands together with the palms facing up to form a bowl.

- Visualize anything that is bugging you or constantly on your mind sitting in the bowl of your hands.

- Take a long inhale through your nose.

- Exhale by blowing the air into your hands, sending your worry far away. Experiment with a short, strong exhale, or a soft and gentle blowing action, and see which feels better to you.

- Sit quietly for a few moments and notice how you feel. Do you feel lighter?

Note for Kids

If your worries remain after trying an exercise such as this one, or keep coming back, it may be a good idea to talk to a parent or trusted teacher about what is on your mind.

WHALE BREATH

What Is Whale Breath and How Does It Help?

Whale Breath is a relaxing breath and body movement that releases lower-back tension by lengthening and gently rotating the spine. Using the breath and gravity, the spine releases into a twist and lengthens as the rest of the body relaxes. Linking movement to breath slows down the breath and deepens it, resulting in greater levels of relaxation.

» *Also good for: relaxation and focus*

 SIMPLE STEPS FOR KIDS

- Lie on your back. Place both feet flat on the floor with the knees pointing up toward the ceiling. Feet can be hip-width distance apart or wider. This is your whale tail!

- Extend the arms out along the floor in a T position. Take a deep breath in through the nose.

- Keep both shoulders relaxed against the floor, drop both knees to the right, and turn your head to look left as you slowly blow the air out through the mouth. This is your whale spout.

- Inhale through the nose as you bring the knees (tail) and head (spout) back to center; exhale through the mouth as you drop the knees to the left and turn your head to the right.

- Repeat for several rounds, gently blowing the air from your whale's spout as you gently swish your tail from side to side.

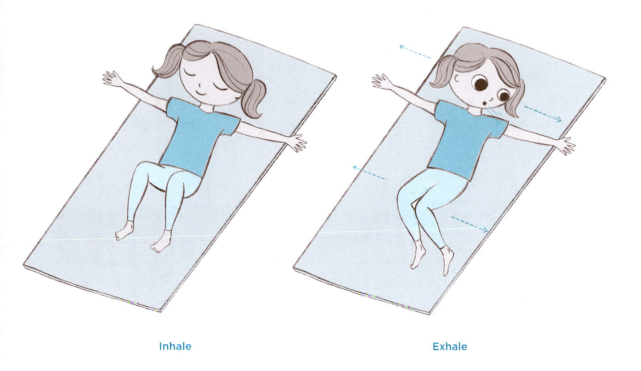

Inhale

Exhale

TIP: *As your child twists, it is important that both shoulders stay in contact with the floor. Your child's knees may not make it all the way to the floor, and that's okay! Eventually gravity, combined with the deep release encouraged by her exhales, will soften any physical resistance and tightness.*

TAP-TAP-TAP

What Is Tap-Tap-Tap?

Tap-Tap-Tap is a self-massage technique that not only feels great but also gets all of the cells in your child's body buzzing, providing the anchor for a meditation that focuses on sensation.

How Does It Help?

Like adults, kids often live inside their heads or focus on everybody and everything around them, without paying too much attention to their own bodies and minds. Self-massage and meditation help them to be in tune with and understand their bodies—allowing them to discover any areas where they may be holding tension that they can then work toward releasing using stretching and breathing techniques or simple awareness. Beyond self-massage, the sensations created when kids use the Tap-Tap-Tap technique make a great focal point for meditation, enhancing body awareness and promoting a deep sense of relaxation.

» *Also good for: focus*

SIMPLE STEPS FOR KIDS

- Begin in a comfortable seated position in a chair or on the floor.
- Using gentle finger pressure, lightly tap the top of your head.
- Move along the back of the head, the sides of the head and temples, and across the forehead.
- Gently tap around the eye sockets, back to the temples, and down the jaw.
- One at a time, squeeze each shoulder with the opposite hand, like you are kneading dough to make bread.

- Fold your hands into soft fists and gently tap across the chest. You can let out some sounds like Tarzan pounding his chest.

- Gently tap the fist down the inside of one arm, tap the palm and the back of hand, and then tap all the way back up the outside of the arm.

- Tap across the chest again to the opposite arm and repeat on that arm.

- With palms flat, gently pat the belly area, then the sides of the torso, and reach around the back and gently pat the kidney area and lower back.

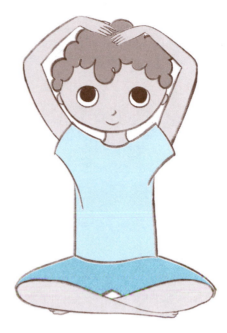

Tap with fingertips

- Starting at the top of one thigh, gently tap your fist down the inside of the leg, tap the sole of the foot, the top of the foot, and all the way back up the outside of the leg. Repeat on the other leg.

- Once finished, gently close your eyes and notice all the sensations you feel in the body. Focus in great detail on each one—tingling, buzzing, and so on—observing all the sensations your massage has created until they fade.

- When you feel ready, slowly open your eyes and notice how good you feel.

PART FOUR

The Chill Zone

TECHNIQUES FOR SUPER RELAXED, HAPPY KIDS

Imagine leaving your smartphone, MP3 player, computer, or tablet on all of the time and never turning it off or recharging it. Eventually, the battery will burn out. Well, kids are no different! The mind and body are both busy machines that work incredibly hard, and, not unlike a computer or smartphone, resting and recharging is key to performing optimally and avoiding burnout.

The exercises presented in The Chill Zone provide the tools and know-how to unplug, reboot, and recharge the mind and body. Removing stimulation while practicing these exercises will provide kids the opportunity to relax and enjoy the benefits of a mini-break from the hustle and bustle of daily life. Reemerging with a sense of calm and well-being, children develop an understanding and appreciation for the value of relaxation, inspiring them to practice on their own.

If your child is just chilling out, is it really meditation? Of course! When practicing progressive relaxation—bringing attention to and relaxing one body part or area at a time—or guided meditation, the mind must remain present. While the focus may be on relaxing and recharging the body, the mind is benefiting as well through single-pointed focus throughout the practice.

Guidelines

Before practicing relaxation or meditation techniques with kids, always do the following:

- Remove any stimuli or potential distractions. Cell phones should be switched off and DO NOT DISTURB signs hung if appropriate.

- Be sure that everybody is comfortable and has anything they may need within reach, such as blankets or pillows.

- Dim the lights and play soft, soothing music.

- Give kids permission to leave during practice to use the bathroom if needed. This way a child won't be uncomfortable or disturb others by asking to go during practice.

- Kids may fall asleep during a particularly long or relaxing practice. Let them know this is natural and they should not feel embarrassed if they do. Falling asleep means they need the rest.

- When rousing a sleeping child, it is important not to startle or frighten them. Use a feather to gently stroke their hands, feet, or face. Be sure to explain this is what you will be doing should they fall asleep before commencing practice and talk to them as you apply the feather strokes—for example, "The magic wake-up feather is gently waking you up now . . . "

TAKE FIVE

What Is Take Five?

Take Five is a breathing technique that acts as a quick fix, helping us breathe and relax, especially during moments of stress. "Take five" is a common expression used when people intend to take a break from a task or job they are doing. In this instance, think of it as a break for your child's mind and body. Kids can Take Five anytime they feel they need it.

How Does It Help?

When we feel nervous, anxious, or stressed, natural reactions are to hold the breath, breathe rapidly, or breathe in uneven and choppy bursts. These reactions only create more stress within the mind and body. Take Five teaches kids to connect with the breath and use it as a tool to steady and calm the mind and body. Sometimes we cannot change or control a situation or experience, but we can control how we react to it. The ability to slow and even out the breath is a fantastic tool, enabling kids to take control of how they respond to stress and tension.

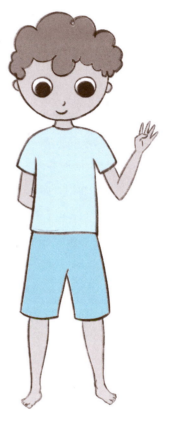

Count to five

» *Also good for: breath control, stress-busting, and focus*

SIMPLE STEPS FOR KIDS

- Hold up your hand, splaying all four fingers and the thumb wide.

- Slowly breathe in to the count of five, curling one finger in at a time as you count off: 1-2-3-4-5.

- Once you reach five, pause, and then slowly breathe out to a count of five, extending one finger at a time back out as you count: 1-2-3-4-5.

- Repeat for several rounds and then return to natural breathing.

- Check in with the rhythm of your natural breath. You should find it is naturally slower and more even after completing just a few rounds of Take Five.

- Observe how you feel—hopefully more centered and calm.

BREATHE IN, BREATHE OUT, RELAX

What Is Breathe In, Breathe Out, Relax?

Breathe In, Breathe Out, Relax is a simple mantra-type breathing exercise kids can practice anywhere and anytime. This technique serves as a quick fix during moments of tension, stress, or anxiety, as well as to calm oneself when excess energy or silliness bubbles within.

How Does It Help?

Immediately drawing attention to the breath, Breathe In, Breathe Out, Relax is a breathing technique that encourages slow and steady breathing, calming the nervous system and disarming the fight-or-flight response—a natural reaction to stressful situations. Breathe In, Breathe Out, Relax is a handy tool kids can access anytime they need it. The simple mantra keeps them connected to the breath and their present actions, removing the focus from anything that may have triggered feelings of stress, anxiety, or worry.

» *Also good for: breath control, stress-busting, and focus*

TIP: *The cue "relax" is a gentle reminder to use each cycle of breath, especially the exhale, to relax; however, feel free to change this to anything that may support your child! For example: "Let go," "I'm safe," or "I'm strong."*

SIMPLE STEPS FOR KIDS

- When you find yourself experiencing a moment of stress or anxiety (or impatience waiting in a long line!), immediately draw your attention to your breath.

- Close your mouth and begin to breathe through your nose.

- Slow and deepen your next inhale, saying the words "Breathe in" to yourself as you feel the ribs expanding in all directions.

- As you breathe out through the nose, slowly and with control say to yourself "Breathe out."

- Once the air is expelled, and before taking your next inhale, say to yourself "Relax."

- Repeat for several rounds until you feel yourself naturally relaxing and taking deeper, slower breaths.

SHINE YOUR LIGHT: A HEART MEDITATION

What Is A Heart Meditation?

A Heart Meditation uses the unique energy of one's heart as a focal point.

How Does It Help?

When learning to meditate, it is helpful to have a focal point to clear one's mind and truly be present. Taking time out to meditate on a daily basis improves productivity and betters your child's ability to focus on tasks. It is also very relaxing: Think of it as a mini-vacation for your child's body and mind. A Heart Meditation is a particularly effective meditation; the heart produces a lot of energy as it works, constantly pumping blood throughout the body, and when kids really focus on it, they can feel that energy.

» *Also good for: focus*

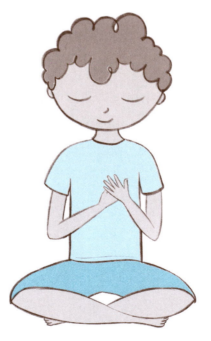

Feel your heart's energy

SIMPLE STEPS FOR KIDS

- Begin in a comfortable seated position. Hold your spine naturally erect, with both feet on the floor if seated in chair.

- Keeping your shoulders and arms relaxed, gently rest your hands on your heart area—slightly left of the chest's center—stacking one hand on top of the other.

- Close your eyes and begin to turn your attention inward. Begin by focusing on the breath, simply observing it entering and leaving the body.

- When you feel ready, move your attention to the area your hands are covering, your heart.

- Silently observe this area, remaining seated with the eyes closed. Do not force yourself to feel anything; just sit and wait for sensations to arise.

- You may feel your heart beating, or sensations such as heat or a vibration or buzz of energy beneath your hands. You may feel an emotion—remember, the heart is not only a muscle pumping blood through our bodies, but also our center for compassion.

- If you feel a strong energy from your heart, radiate it out to other areas of your body. That is, start with the energy you feel in the center of your chest and "grow" it so you eventually feel that energy spreading throughout your entire body.

- Sit here for five to ten minutes, enjoying the energy from your heart. Feel it shine and spread throughout your body.

- Gently release your hands to your lap and take several slow, deep breaths before gradually opening your eyes.

MAGIC FEATHER MEDITATION

What Is Magic Feather Meditation?

Magic Feather Meditation is a relaxation technique that uses light feather strokes to calm and relax the body and mind.

How Does It Help?

Light feather strokes soothe and calm the nervous system and gently stimulate the sensory system, helping with body awareness and proprioception (the sense of where the physical body is positioned or located in space). Most people find this exercise soothing and relaxing—like magic!

» *Also good for: focus, stress-busting, and energy equalizing*

TIP: *Use short, upward strokes to energize, and long, downward strokes to calm.*

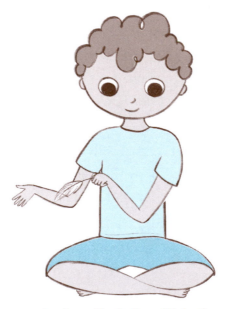

Apply gentle strokes with feather

SIMPLE STEPS FOR KIDS

Magic Feather Meditation is best done partnered up with a friend; however, it can be adapted as a self-massage/meditation technique.

Partner Activity

- One partner lies comfortably on the floor with eyes gently closed. He takes a few deep inhales and exhales before letting go and allowing the breath to be natural and the body to be relaxed, fully supported by the floor.

- The second person, using a feather, gently applies soft strokes along the arms, legs, and face, gently tracing the jawline, temples, forehead, bridge of nose, and neck (making sure to avoid the eyes and the inside of the ears and nose).

- Encourage the person applying the feather strokes to use this exercise as a meditation, staying focused and present, and observing any subtle responses in their partner. Switch roles.

Individual Meditation/Self-Massage

Begin in a comfortable seated position. Close your eyes and take a few deep inhales and exhales to feel centered and present. Using a feather, gently begin to apply soft strokes to your body. Try out different pressures and movements, noticing how each one makes you feel and which areas of the body you are drawn to—are you holding tension in that particular area? Or, follow this simple routine:

- Begin with light feather strokes on the back of the hand and fingers. Move to the palm, then along the arm, all the way to the shoulder (be sure to cover entire arm, back and front, with light feathery strokes). Repeat with other arm.

- Gently sweep the feather along the jawline and temples, across the forehead, down the bridge of the nose, over and under the chin, and on the neck. (Sweep the sides and back of the neck if your feather can reach).

- Sweep down one leg, all the way to the foot (be sure to cover the entire leg, back and front).

- Sweep the top of the foot and ankle, and then the sole of the foot with the feather. Repeat on the other side.

No Feather? No Problem!

Kids can use their fingertips! Apply very soft, gentle strokes by lightly dragging the fingertips in an upward or downward motion, barely touching the body.

WAX MUSEUM

What is Wax Museum?

Wax Museum is a fun relaxation technique during which kids start out as stiff as a wax sculpture, and then slowly melt in the sun into a puddle of soft, gooey wax.

How Does It Help?

Wax Museum is a meditative relaxation technique that systematically relaxes the physical body and the mind. It is helpful for anxiety, insomnia, and general physical or mental fatigue.

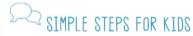 SIMPLE STEPS FOR KIDS

- Begin by lying on the floor, your bed, or a sofa.
- Stretch your arms up overhead; stretch out the fingers and point the toes. Make your body as long as you can.
- Imagine you are a wax sculpture, like those you see at a wax museum.
- Release the stretch, resting the arms alongside the torso, and allow the feet to fall apart.
- Imagine your entire body is sculpted from wax.
- Imagine a bright sun warming your entire body.
- As your body begins to warm, imagine the wax softening.
- Beginning at the top of your head, mentally scan your way slowly down the entire body and imagine each part softening and melting.
- Once you visit each area of the body independently, then reconnect the body as a whole and imagine it melted on the floor—one large piece of soft and gooey wax, warm from the sun. Rest here for five to ten minutes.

SQUEEZE AND RELEASE

What Is Squeeze and Release?

Squeeze and Release is a relaxation technique where one systematically contracts the muscles in the body before releasing and relaxing them.

How Does It Help?

Squeeze and Release relaxes the entire physical body—especially areas where kids may be holding tension—preparing the body for sleep, relaxation, or rest. This is a great technique to use before going to bed or before beginning a meditation.

» *Also good for: stress-busting and energy equalizing*

 SIMPLE STEPS FOR KIDS

- Begin in a restful position lying on your back.

- Curl the toes on both feet and release. Repeat several times.

- Flex and point the feet and then rotate the ankles in both directions.

- Resting the legs on the floor, flex the toes toward your nose, engaging the muscles in both legs. Relax and repeat several times.

- Hug the knees into the chest and squeeze them tightly. Rock gently from side to side. Make small circles with the knees in both directions. Release and relax the legs along the floor.

- Stretch both arms overhead and point the toes away from the body, giving the entire body a stretch.

- Clench and release the fists of both hands several times. Rest the arms alongside the torso and relax the feet, allowing them to fall open.

- Wrap your arms across your torso and give yourself a big hug, squeezing the shoulders. Release.

- Stretch the mouth open wide in a huge yawn. Release and repeat.

- Squeeze the eyes closed. Release and repeat.

- Hug the knees into the chest and squeeze them tightly. Tuck the chin toward the chest and curl into a small ball. Squeeze everything in as tightly as possible—face, ears, eyes, and toes— for a count of 1-2-3. Release.

- Imagine you are a huge puddle of water as you fully release and spread out on the floor, taking as much space as you need. Relax in this position for five to ten minutes.

BODY SCAN

What Is Body Scan?

Body Scan is a relaxation technique for the mind and body.

How Does It Help?

Mentally scanning the entire body by visiting one area at a time requires presence and focus, which has a deeply meditative and relaxing effect on the mind and the body. Body Scan is also a valuable tool that helps kids recognize areas in the body where they hold tension, giving them the option to consciously relax these areas while practicing, as well as providing an awareness of any tension building in these areas on a daily basis. When they become aware of areas or "hot spots" where they carry tension, they can then work to release them.

» *Also good for: focus*

TIPS:

- *If your child notices tension somewhere, he can breathe deeply and visualize that area, expanding as he inhales and relaxing as he exhales.*

- *Make this activity fun! Have your child imagine a magic laser light glowing, warming, and relaxing each area as he visits it. Or, he can imagine a colorful feather gently sweeping each area, calming and relaxing him with light feathery strokes.*

SIMPLE STEPS FOR KIDS

- Begin in a comfortable position—preferably lying on your back. If this is not possible, then sit comfortably in a chair, both feet in contact with the floor, spine naturally erect, shoulders and arms relaxed, and hands resting in your lap.

- Close your eyes and begin to observe the natural rhythm of your breath, following each inhale and exhale. Let go of any thoughts as you do so.

- Once you feel ready to begin, move your attention through the body. Pause at each area, noting any sensation that arises and, even if that area feels relaxed, see if you can consciously relax it even more. Once that area feels completely relaxed, move on to the next point. Use the following as a guide, focusing on each of these areas:

  1. Top of the head: Notice every detail, including the scalp and hair.
  2. Back of the head: Notice which areas contact the floor or pillow.
  3. Forehead and temples
  4. Eyes: Pay attention to the eyelashes and eyebrows too.
  5. Nose
  6. Jaw: Include the mouth, teeth, and tongue.
  7. Throat
  8. Neck (front and back)
  9. Collarbones
  10. Shoulders

11. Right arm and hand: Scan the right upper arm, elbow, and forearm, followed by the right hand—its palm, each finger, and thumb.

12. Chest and torso

13. Left arm and hand: Scan the left upper arm, elbow, and forearm, followed by the left hand—its palm, each finger, and thumb.

14. Upper back: Notice which areas are in contact with the floor or pillow.

15. Abdomen

16. Hips: Notice which areas are in contact with the floor or pillow.

17. Lower back: Allow the lower back area to soften into the support of the pillow or floor beneath you.

18. Right leg: Scan the front and back of the thigh, followed by the knee, calf, and lower leg, and the right foot, including each toe.

19. Left leg: Scan the front and back of the thigh, followed by the knee, calf, and lower leg, and the left foot, including each toe.

20. Connect the whole body together. Imagine the entire body, deeply relaxed.

- Breathe and soak in the sensations of a completely relaxed body. Stay here for at least five to ten minutes, or longer if needed.

MAGIC CARPET RIDE

What Is Magic Carpet Ride?

Magic Carpet Ride is a guided relaxation technique often used in kids' yoga classes, but this does not mean it is just for kids! Adults and teens also enjoy—and *benefit* from—the freedom of choosing and imagining a journey to a special place of their own.

How Does It Help?

Magic Carpet Ride gives kids the power to choose, dream, imagine, escape, and let go. Since kids are creating this relaxing journey in their minds, they are free to keep it to themselves or share it with others once they finish. It is a great exercise that provides a safe haven kids can visit anytime they feel the need to take a break from their everyday lives.

TIP: *Teachers: When guiding a group or a class, gently suggest students imagine and answer your questions silently rather than speaking aloud. You may need to keep gently reminding them, or pose your suggestions in a way that encourages silent reflection, such as "Now in your mind, imagine what color your magic carpet is" . . . or, "Remember, this is your own special place, so keep it a secret in your mind as you land your magic carpet there."*

SIMPLE STEPS FOR KIDS

- Begin in a comfortable resting position, preferably on your back. (You can sit if lying down is uncomfortable for any reason.)

- Turn down the lights and use blankets and pillows to help you relax and be as comfortable as possible.

- Gently close the eyes and leave them closed for the duration of this exercise.

- Take a few deep breaths as you scan your body from head to toe to be sure it is relaxed and loose.

- Imagine the surface beneath you is a beautiful magic carpet. Envision every detail: What color is it? Does it have any patterns or embellishments? What fabric is it made from? What texture is it? This is *your* magic carpet, so make it anything you want.

- Feel your magic carpet beneath you, holding you, supporting you, and keeping you safe. The magic carpet begins to gently lift you off the floor and out of the room, light as a feather yet fully supported.

- Feel the wind lightly caress your face and body as your magic carpet slowly glides over the city where you began this journey. Drifting past the clouds, your magic carpet lifts you up, higher and higher, over the treetops. Listen to the birds in the trees chirping hello to you as you float by.

- Passing by clouds, you reach out to touch their billowy softness. Feel the wind gently caress you, the soft clouds touching you as you float by, fully supported, safe and secure on your beautiful magic carpet.

- Drift toward your special, soothing place. This can be anywhere: a park, the beach, a forest, another city or country, a different planet, or a magical land—anywhere you want to go that feels special to you! Your magic carpet has the ability to travel anywhere you can imagine—just picture a place in your mind and it will take you there.

- Feel the wind brush your face as your magic carpet gently lowers you down to your imagined place.

- Notice how it feels to be in this special spot. Listen to the sounds around you. What do you hear? What does it smell like? Who is here with you? You are safe and secure, enjoying your own happy place. Know you can come here anytime you like . . . it belongs to you.

- Stay as long as you like, enjoying all the sensations of being here. When you are ready to return, take one last look around. Wave goodbye to all the people, animals, and/or creatures, and know you can visit them again anytime you like.

- Feel your magic carpet lift you up, floating up ever so slowly to the sky. Touch the soft, fluffy clouds as you drift by and feel the breeze on your skin as your magic carpet makes its way back to where you began this journey. Feel the warm sun shining on your face as you float in the sky, ever so safely, on your beautiful magic carpet. Hear the birds chirping, "Hello! Welcome back!" as you sail over the treetops and then, finally, softly land back where you began.

- Rest here as long as you like, taking in all of the sensations and remembering the details of your amazing journey.

- Once you feel ready, slowly sit up. If you like, you can share your experience with a friend, write a journal entry, or draw a picture of your adventure.

INK BATH

What Is Ink Bath?

Ink Bath is a body-awareness exercise that focuses on the physical body while engaging the imagination.

How Does It Help?

Being fully aware and present in the body is a form of meditation. Meditation allows kids' minds and bodies to have a mini-break from their busy daily lives, leaving them feeling calm and relaxed and giving them the ability to be more focused and get things done!

» *Also good for: focus*

 SIMPLE STEPS FOR KIDS

Ink Bath can be practiced lying down or seated. Seated is preferable if you want to quickly refocus or take a true "mini" break; lying down is beneficial when you want to relax for a little bit longer.

- Gently close your eyes and take a few deep breaths to feel centered.

- Imagine your favorite color; now imagine a bath filled with ink the exact shade of your favorite color.

- Keep your eyes closed and imagine taking a bath, soaking in your favorite color.

- Visualize your entire body covered in your favorite color ink; now imagine returning to the floor or your chair.

- Slowly and carefully scan your body, noticing which areas make contact with the floor (or chair), and imagine the stamp or impression your body is making. Remember some parts of your body will be making full contact, while other areas will barely touch, and some won't make contact with the floor or chair at all—leaving a series of colored shapes or imprints.

- Once you have scanned your entire body and imagined all the different shapes it would make on the floor or chair, begin to connect the image—that is, imagine your inky impression as a whole, like a piece of art.

- Is your impression the same on both sides, or different? What shapes are there? Are they all connected or are there spaces and gaps in between? Are there heavy and dark areas and other areas with very light impressions, barely touching?

- When you feel ready, gently open your eyes. Can you still feel the areas where your body makes contact with the floor or chair? Do you feel more aware of your body? More present?

SIXTY-ONE–POINT MEDITATION

What Is Sixty-One–Point Meditation and How Does It Help?

The Sixty-One–Point Meditation exercise can be practiced in two ways:

- Lying down, it serves as a deep relaxation exercise.

- In a seated position, it serves as a concentration/focus exercise.

» Also good for: focus

SIMPLE STEPS FOR KIDS

- Refer to the attached diagram for the location of each of the sixty-one points on the body. (Note: It will take several practice sessions before you begin to memorize the points, enabling you to flow seamlessly through this meditation.)

- Begin in a comfortable position, either seated or lying on the floor. Set yourself up with blankets, pillows, or whatever you need to be sure you are comfortable.

- Relax the body as you begin to deepen the breath and settle in.

- When you feel ready to begin, shift your focus to the first point on the diagram.

- Slowly move through the sequence, mentally traveling from one point on the body to the next, using one of the following focus tips, until you reach the sixty-first point.

  - ＊ FOCUS: Slowly move from one point to the next, focusing all your attention on each point as if it were the only part of your body.

* BREATHE: Settle on each point and remain focused on it as you breathe in and out for a count of breaths, completing the same number of breath cycles at each point. For example, count one to five full breath cycles at each point. Visualize the breath entering and exiting the body through each point on which you are focused.

* COUNT: Visit each point and name it by its number as you focus on it. For example, count "one," "two," "three," . . . "fifty-nine," "sixty," "sixty-one" as you visit each point.

* VISUALIZE: Envision a color saturating each point. Slowly work your way from point to point, visualizing that area of the body being bathed in a color of your choosing. For example, you may choose blue, a calming color. It may also be helpful to visualize a shape, such as a blue star or circle, pulsing at each point.

• Once you have visited each of the sixty-one points, continue to sit or lie in a relaxed state for as long as you need.

TIPS:

• *Help your child fully engage in the exercise without referring to the chart by creating a recording of the points or by reading them to your child during practice.*

• *Understand that in this exercise, some areas of the body are visited multiple times. This is to slow the pace and mindfully move through the body, stopping at each point along the way. For example, when journeying back from a distal area, such as the fingertips, instead of rushing back to the shoulder, the mind is guided to revisit the wrist and elbow to slow its journey and further relax the arm.*

SIXTY-ONE-POINT MEDITATION

1. Center of forehead	22. Left pinky finger
2. Base of front of neck	23. Left wrist
3. Right shoulder	24. Left elbow
4. Right elbow	25. Left shoulder
5. Right wrist	26. Base of front of neck
6. Right thumb	27. Center of chest
7. Right index finger	28. Right side of chest
8. Right middle finger	29. Center of chest
9. Right ring finger	30. Left side of chest
10. Right pinky finger	31. Center of chest
11. Right wrist	32. Belly button
12. Right elbow	33. Lower belly
13. Right shoulder	34. Right hip
14. Base of front of neck	35. Right knee
15. Left shoulder	36. Right ankle
16. Left elbow	37. Right big toe
17. Left wrist	38. Right second toe
18. Left thumb	39. Right third toe
19. Left index finger	40. Right fourth toe
20. Left middle finger	41. Right little toe
21. Left ring finger	42. Right ankle

43. Right knee

44. Right hip

45. Lower belly

46. Left hip

47. Left knee

48. Left ankle

49. Left big toe

50. Left second toe

51. Left third toe

52. Left fourth toe

53. Left little toe

54. Left ankle

55. Left knee

56. Left hip

57. Lower belly

58. Belly button

59. Center of chest

60. Base of front of neck

61. Center of forehead

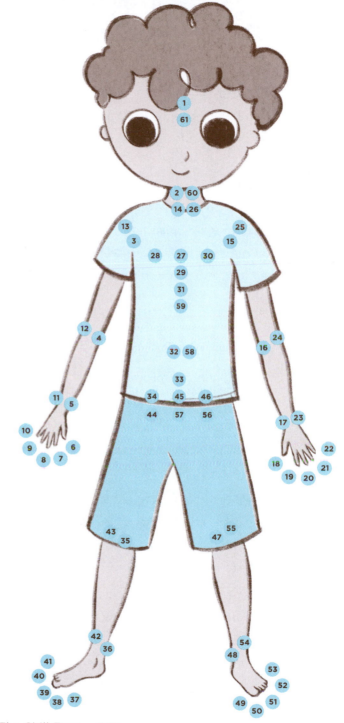

THE BIG CHILLAX

What Is the BIG Chillax?

The BIG Chillax is exactly as it sounds: a BIG moment to do nothing but chill and relax, giving kids' bodies and minds the BIG rest they deserve.

How Does It Help?

Our bodies are constantly on the go, and our minds are often chatting away incessantly, creating stories, planning, remembering, and more. Turning everything off and recharging not only makes kids feel good but also gives them more energy to do the things they love and do them well.

 SIMPLE STEPS FOR KIDS

- Begin in a comfortable position lying on the floor.

- Prop a pillow under the knees to release any pressure from the lower back and a pillow under the head for comfort. Your body temperature drops when you relax, so keep a blanket close by in case you need it.

- Allow your feet to fall apart and the arms to rest alongside the torso, with the palms facing up. Gently close your eyes and take a few deep inhales and exhales before allowing the breath to fall into its natural rhythm.

- Let go. Allow your body to "let go" and be fully supported by the floor and pillows. Allow the mind to release any thoughts. This part will not be easy! The mind will always want to think, chat, and talk—it is constantly running a commentary. The trick is to let your mind do its thing without encouraging it by attaching to any of those thoughts. If you find yourself trailing along a thought, simply stop and detach yourself from it. Do this each time the mind tries to get your attention. Let it go.

- The aim of this exercise is to stop doing and simply be. Be calm. Be still. Be relaxed. Let go. Do nothing. Chill. Relax. Chillax.

- Remain in this relaxed state for ten to thirty minutes. When it is time to finish, do so slowly. Gently rouse the mind and body by deepening your breath, and slowly move the tongue around in the mouth. Gently wiggle your fingers and toes and then roll your wrists and ankles.

- When you feel ready, draw the knees in toward your chest and roll onto one side into the fetal position. Rest here for a moment before gently using your arms to press yourself up into a comfortable seated position.

- Sit with the eyes closed for a few moments and enjoy the sensations of relaxation.

TIP: *To really enjoy the benefits of the BIG Chillax, be sure to make your child as comfortable as possible: Dim the lights, close the shades, play soothing music, and use pillows, blankets, and eye pillows.*

OCEAN DRIFT

What Is Ocean Drift and How Does It Help?

Ocean Drift is an auditory meditation technique that relaxes the mind and body.

What Do You Need?

- Comfortable place to lie still and relax

- Ocean sounds audio track

- Sound system to play track

- Pillows, blankets, and bolsters as needed for comfort

TIP: *Ocean sounds audio tracks are available on iTunes and other websites. You may also find such tracks on relaxation CDs available at local music stores, health food stores, or department stores. If your child doesn't enjoy ocean sounds, you can substitute any track your child finds soothing and relaxing—forest sounds, singing birds, rushing water, and the like.*

Getting Started

- Set up the sound system to "loop" the ocean sounds audio track for as long as your child would like to enjoy this meditation/relaxation exercise.

- Play track and turn the lights off or down while your child gets comfortable.

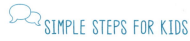

SIMPLE STEPS FOR KIDS

- Lie on your back. Set yourself up with any props necessary for your comfort, such as pillows or blankets.

- Take several deep breaths as your body releases onto the floor. Allow the mind to let go of any thoughts as you settle in and relax.

- Let the body go completely, allowing the floor to fully support it.

- Shift your attention to the sounds of the ocean's waves filling the room.

- Allow the waves to wash over you, each wave bringing a new and deeper sense of relaxation to your body and mind. Release any tension with each receding wave. Allow the ocean to ebb and flow, maintaining a focus on the sounds.

- When you're ready to end the meditation, rest a little longer without the music, enjoying the benefits of this exercise before slowly sitting up.

SLEEPING MOUSE

What Is Sleeping Mouse?

Sleeping Mouse is a restorative body posture, meaning there is no physical effort required. Also known as child's pose or rock pose, Sleeping Mouse is a resting posture that allows the body and mind to relax.

How Does It Help?

Sleeping Mouse releases tension in the back, shoulders, and chest while gently lengthening and stretching the spine, as well as stretching the hips, thighs, and ankles. It alleviates stress and anxiety, calming the mind and body, and is highly recommended when your child is feeling overwhelmed. This technique is also helpful when your child is feeling excitable, as it is stabilizing and grounding.

» *Also good for: focus, stress-busting, and energy equalizing*

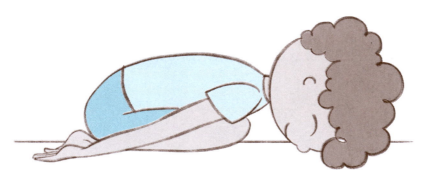

Quiet as a mouse

SIMPLE STEPS FOR KIDS

- Start on your knees and sit back on your heels.
- Slowly fold the upper body forward so that your torso rests on your thighs.
- Stack your fists and rest your forehead on them. Breathe.
- Gently move your fists and allow your forehead to rest on the floor.
- Rest your arms alongside your torso and legs, with the palms facing up. Breathe deeply and rest here for as long as you like.
- To move out of Sleeping Mouse, slowly stretch your arms in front of you on the floor and walk the hands in toward the body as you rise to a seated position.

TIP: *If you experience pain in your knees, or if you have a knee injury, then simply lie on your back and hug your knees in toward your chest. Keep your head and shoulders resting on the floor and close your eyes. Breathe slowly.*

RAINBOW, RAINBOW MEDITATION

What Is Rainbow, Rainbow Meditation?

Rainbow, Rainbow Meditation is a visualization technique that draws on nature and color therapy to help kids feel relaxed, vibrant, and confident.

How Does It Help?

Color therapy is based on the theory that colors can trigger certain psychological or emotional states. For example, blue is thought to be calming, while yellow is perceived as energizing. As kids relax in your Rainbow, Rainbow Meditation, they will be guided to visualize the different colors of the rainbow and the positive mind states each color represents. After this meditation, your child should feel radiant and fabulous—just like a rainbow!

 SIMPLE STEPS FOR KIDS

- Begin in a comfortable position lying on the floor.

- Prop a pillow under the knees to release any pressure on the lower back and a pillow under the head for comfort. Your body temperature drops when you relax, so keep a blanket close by in case you need it.

- Allow the feet to fall apart and the arms to rest alongside the torso, with the palms facing up. Gently close your eyes and take a few deep inhales and exhales before allowing the breath to fall into its natural rhythm.

- Imagine floating on a soft billowy cloud, light as a feather yet fully supported.

- Visualize the arc of a beautiful rainbow spreading above you, beginning at your toes and stretching up over your body to your head.
- Imagine each color bathing you from your toes to your head and back again, connecting your whole body beneath the image of a rainbow. As you envision each color, soak up all of the positive qualities each color brings:

RED: *POWER and STRENGTH*

ORANGE: *JOY and CREATIVITY*

YELLOW: *SUNSHINE and CONFIDENCE*

GREEN: *LOVING KINDNESS*

BLUE: *HONESTY*

INDIGO: *INTUITION*

VIOLET: *LOYALTY and WISDOM*

- Take your time to truly feel and experience each color and its qualities before moving on to the next.
- Relax and rest under your completed rainbow, soaking in its vibrant energy for as long as you like.

CROCODILE

What Is Crocodile?

Crocodile is a restorative body posture that uses props rather than muscle engagement to support the body and maintain the posture, allowing the body to relax fully.

How Does It Help?

Crocodile is a grounding posture, meaning the body and mind will feel anchored and connected to the present moment rather than scattered and/or anxious. It is calming and relaxing.

» Also good for: focus and stress-busting

What Do You Need?

- A bolster (or folded-up blanket or pillow)
- A yoga block

No Yoga Block? No Problem!

If you do not have a yoga block, then you can stack your hands or fists on top of one another and rest your forehead on top.

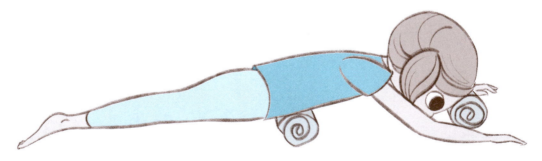

Sink deeper with each exhale

SIMPLE STEPS FOR KIDS

- Lie facedown on your belly, placing the bolster (or folded blanket) under your rib cage.

- Place a yoga block or rolled-up blanket under your forehead.

- Relax your arms and legs completely, allowing the body to be fully supported by the props and the floor.

- Breathe deeply, feeling the belly expand and release against the floor.

- Allow yourself to be heavy; imagine sinking deeper into the floor with each exhale.

- Stay in this deeply relaxing pose for five to ten minutes.

PART FIVE

Connect

PLAYFUL WAYS TO INTRODUCE WELLNESS TO PARTNERS AND/OR SMALL GROUPS

While time for quiet reflection is important, kids also benefit from connecting to others in playful and healthy ways. Many of the techniques featured in this book can be practiced in groups; however, the techniques in this part of the book were specifically designed to teach kids meditation and wellness skills while fostering teamwork, cooperation, communication, and social awareness—all while having fun! Working with others, kids develop essential social skills and improve the ability to cultivate and maintain relationships.

Tips for Parents

This section is not just for kids to play and connect with their friends but a great way to encourage siblings to collaborate, play and learn together, and build strong, healthy relationships.

Many parents tell me they want to learn how to be more playful with their kids. The following activities are a wonderful opportunity to do just that—you'll strengthen your bond with your child and learn how to meditate in a fun and lighthearted way too.

Tips for Teachers

Many of the techniques presented in this book are effective tools to break up the academic day and benefit your students by increasing their ability to focus, process, and retain information. Fun, active classroom breaks get kids out of their seats and heads, and into their bodies to release pent-up tension and find their "happy place."

Accessing the following activities in small groups or with partners has the additional benefit of cultivating peer connection through play, resulting in a healthy social environment in your class. Who doesn't want a classroom full of happy, joyful, focused kids who get along with each other?

FEEL THE VIBRATION

What Is Feel the Vibration?

Feel the Vibration is a fun technique that teaches kids how they can use their breath and body in different ways to make certain sounds.

How Does It Help?

Developing an awareness of the breath and our ability to control it is an important aspect of the mind–body connection. This exercise demonstrates that just as kids can make sounds at will, they have the ability to bring a sense of relaxation and calm to their bodies and minds by using their breath.

» *Also good for: breath control, focus, stress-busting, and energy equalizing*

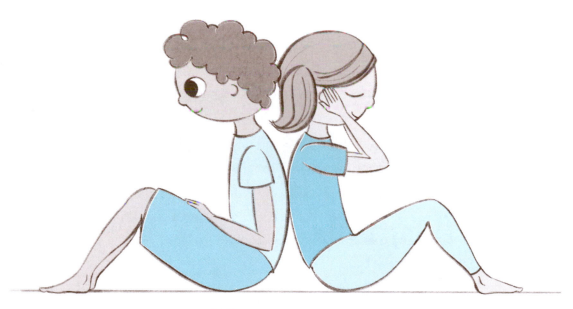

Feel your partner's vibration

SIMPLE STEPS FOR KIDS

- Begin in a comfortable seated position, spine naturally erect. Place your feet flat on the floor, relax your shoulders and arms, and rest your hands in your lap.

- Begin humming an "mmmm" sound. Notice where you feel it most (for this sound, it will most likely be the lips and mouth).

- Continue making the sound and scan the body for other areas the sound is affecting, such as the throat or even farther down in the abdominal area. For example, you may feel the belly pulling in as you make the "mmmm" sound.

- Play around with different sounds and examine each one. Notice where you feel it in the body the most, followed by the more subtle areas.

- As you try out different sounds, ask yourself questions about each one. Where does the sound originate? Where does it end? What muscles engage? Do any relax? How does each sound differ from the others? Are some similar in regard to their effect on the body?

- Now sit back-to-back with a friend or partner. Notice how each sound feels coming from a different person.

- Play a game: Cover your ears with your hands and see if you can guess which sound your partner is making based on the vibration and movement you feel coming from her body. Switch and take turns.

Some Sounds to Try

Short sounds originate in the core of the body and engage the diaphragm to "push" out the air to make the sound. The breath (and sound) comes out in a short burst of energy. This kind of breath is great to release any pent-up energy or stress; it can also energize kids when they are feeling sluggish.

Long sounds tend to originate from the chest and require an extended, smooth exhale to carry them along. The body feels like a tire deflating when making long sounds, and doing so can help kids to relax mentally and physically.

LONG: "aaah," "vvvv," "ohhh," "aaay," "eeee," "iiii," "oooo," "yoou," "ssss," "zzzz," "sssh," "hmmm," "laaa"

SHORT: "hah," "uh," "ugh," "the," "ba," "pa," "la," "do," "doh," "ga," "car"

TIP: *This fun exercise is a fabulous way to demonstrate just how important the breath is! Beyond the function of breathing for survival, breath is a tool for self-regulation, feeling great, and, as kids will recognize from this technique, creating and vocalizing sounds. Without the breath, they would not be able to talk!*

PEOPLE-POWERED PLANE

What Is People-Powered Plane?

Exploring the breath is fun, especially when kids do it with their friends. People-Powered Plane is a game played with a small group of friends that offers the many benefits of deep breathing and linking movement to breath.

How Does It Help?

Working together is teamwork. Flying a "plane" while breathing in unison teaches kids that *together* they can do anything! The physical movements of People-Powered Plane teach coordination while creating space in the torso to allow for deeper breathing.

» *Also good for: breath control, focus, and stress-busting*

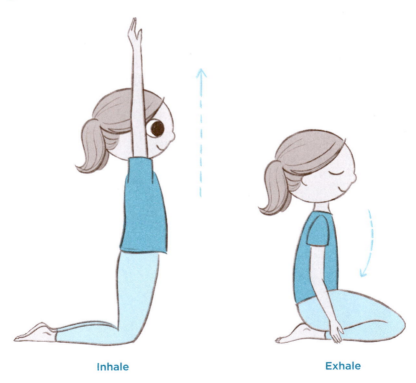

Inhale   Exhale

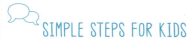

SIMPLE STEPS FOR KIDS

- Sit on the knees, one person behind the other in a row, all facing the same direction.

- Inhale together, flapping your arms in a gentle up-and-down motion as you slowly rise to stand on your knees. At the top of your inhale, you should be standing on your knees with your arms stretched up overhead.

- Exhale together, flapping your arms in a gentle up-and-down motion as you slowly lower to sit back on your heels. At the end of your exhale, you should be kneeling, sitting on your heels, with your arms resting by your side.

- You've now completed one round. Repeat up to five full rounds of in breaths and out breaths.

TIP: *In the beginning, kids may find it difficult to time their own inhales and exhales with those of their friends. This is okay—we all breathe differently. Advise kids to do their best and follow their own breath, without forcing or straining it. Eventually, they will fall into a rhythm with their friends where they are all breathing—and flying—at a similar pace.*

AIR SOCCER

What Is Air Soccer

Air Soccer is a fun game that can be played with friends. It demonstrates how our breath can work in different ways to benefit our health and feelings.

What Do You Need?

- Straws (thick smoothie straws or regular drinking straws)
- Pom-poms, ping-pong balls, or balled-up tissue paper
- Shoe boxes or small- or medium-size boxes (empty, no lids)
- Yoga mat (optional)

» Also good for: breath control

TIP: *The aim is to have control over the direction the pom-pom rolls. Short bursts of breath will send it flying, but players won't have control. Deep inhales with long, controlled exhales will help direct the ball toward the goals and away from the opposition team. Ask kids how breathing this way makes them feel.*

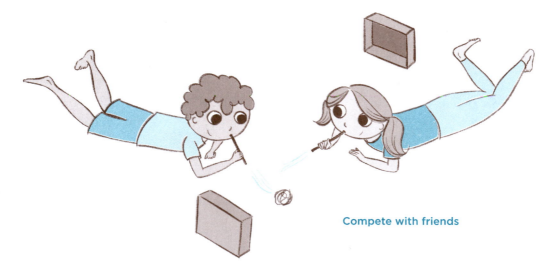

Compete with friends

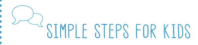 SIMPLE STEPS FOR KIDS

ONE PLAYER

- Lay a shoebox on its side with the open part facing in. Set it at one end of yoga mat or room; this is your "goal."

- Lie on your belly at the other end of the yoga mat or room. Have a straw and pom-pom (or Ping-Pong ball or balled-up tissue paper) with you.

- Gently blow into the straw to move your pom-pom down the mat and into the goal. Play against yourself and see if you can get the ball into the goal with the least amount of breaths. Challenge yourself by placing the goal farther away from your starting point each time.

TWO OR MORE PLAYERS

- Set up goals at each end of floor area and allocate one goal to each team.

- Pass the pom-pom back and forth between players.

- Work together with your teammates to score goals and to stop the opposing team from scoring goals.

- The team with the most goals after a certain time period is declared the winning team. (To avoid too much chaos, allocate one area of the playing field per player, including a goalie for each team. If there are only two players, they may cover the full area.)

GOLF

What Is Golf and How Does It Help?

A variation of the breath game Air Soccer (page 168), Golf is a fun way to learn about the breath and train the body to breathe fully and deeply. This game focuses on lengthening the out breath (or exhale), something players will need to score a hole in one! Golf benefits its players by slowing down the breath, calming the nervous system, and cultivating awareness of the breath and how it can consciously be changed to benefit a person's body (and golf score!).

» *Also good for: breath control*

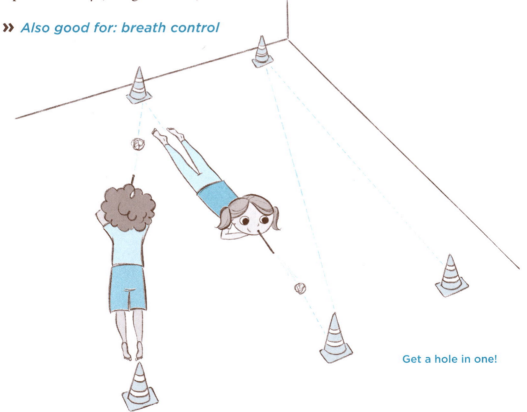

Get a hole in one!

TIP: *Teachers: Break larger classes into smaller groups of up to five players to make the game more manageable.*

What Do You Need?

- A clear floor space, or several yoga mats lined up side by side to create one large surface area

- Beanbags or cones to use as markers

- Straws (bendy ones are easier for kids to maneuver at floor-level)

- Pom-poms or ping-pong balls (balled-up tissue can be used if you don't have pom-poms or ping-pong balls)

 SIMPLE STEPS FOR KIDS

- Set markers in a zigzag pattern on the floor area.

- Player One moves his ball or pom-pom toward the first marker by blowing air through a straw.

- Once Player One passes the first marker, Player Two can begin. (Players move toward each marker after the players in front of them have passed it.)

- The object is for each player to count how many times he blows the ball between markers, and to work toward getting the ball from one marker to the next using one breath—a hole in one!

- While golfers play independently, navigating the course several times and trying to improve their own score, they must remain aware and respectful of others on the course, and communicate effectively so only one player at a time is teeing off and moving between holes—not unlike a real golf course. Social interaction occurs between golfers when they arrive at a busy tee-off point and need to wait their turn.

THE *SSHH* GAME

What Is The *Sshh* Game?

The *Sshh* Game is a fun present-moment awareness exercise that is easy for kids of all ages to play.

How Does It Help?

Present-moment awareness is a great tool to access when your child needs to focus or concentrate. A form of meditation, it is also helpful if he finds himself caught up in thoughts that are not helpful, or at times when he has trouble falling asleep.

» Also good for: focus

 SIMPLE STEPS FOR KIDS

This game can be played in a group or individually.

GROUP

- Begin sitting comfortably in a circle. (Large groups can be broken up into several smaller groups.)
- Center the group by doing a couple of rounds of Balloon Breath (see page 62).
- Determine an order or direction for each member of the circle to take his or her turn.
- Each person begins her turn by saying "Sshh . . . " The rest of the group remains quiet. Once the person feels and then acknowledges a sensation (see What to Do, at right), the next person takes a turn.

INDIVIDUAL

- Begin in a comfortable seated position.

- Close the eyes, take a few deep inhales and exhales until you feel centered, and follow What to Do below.

WHAT TO DO

- Sit quietly and wait until you sense something, such as a smell, taste, sound, or other sensation.

- When you do, say "Sshh . . . " and then "I can feel . . . " or "I can smell . . . " or "I can hear . . . " or whatever expresses the sensation you are experiencing. For example, "Sshh . . . I can feel a breeze on my arm" or "Sshh . . . I can hear a bird singing" or "Sshh . . . I can feel my own heart beating" or "Sshh . . . I can hear a plane flying by."

- Sometimes you may not hear, feel, smell, or taste anything. Just sit quietly and wait until you do. The more quietly you sit, the more likely you are to notice things.

TIP: *Teachers: The "Sshh," or quiet component necessary to play this game, makes it effective in quieting and calming a class that has become rowdy.*

SCARVES

What Is Scarves and How Does It Help?

Scarves is a fun mirroring game that can be played in partners or groups. An active meditation, it encourages slow, fluid physical movements and a quiet, focused mind to play. In addition to the benefits of meditation—a clear, calm, and focused mind—this activity develops coordination skills and balance, while fostering teamwork and intuition.

» *Also good for: focus and stress-busting*

What Do You Need?

- One colorful silk scarf per child

SIMPLE STEPS FOR KIDS

- Begin with partners facing each other, one child elected as leader. If children are in small groups, begin with one child facing each group as the leader.

- The leader slowly moves his scarf around in slow and fluid movements. His partner or group must follow, mirroring his moves, trying to match the leader's movements and speed.

- Leaders are encouraged to keep movements slow and intentional. This is more challenging to mirror than fast, jerky movements and requires greater presence.

- After working with the same leader for a while, players may notice that they begin to guess what the leader's next move will be, naturally moving with him without thinking too much about it. This is known as intuition.

Discussion

After playing Scarves, discuss with players how they felt while playing. Did they find it easy to focus on the scarf and the leader's movements? Or were they easily distracted? Did any players experience their intuition coming into play? If so, discuss intuition: what it is and how it can play a role in other areas of their lives.

More Ways to Play

Scarves can be played as a game of elimination. The child caught not mirroring a move exactly is "out." In the case of a group activity, one player will be eliminated from each round until only one remains and is declared the winner. In the case of a partner activity, the person who is not "out" gets a point; roles are then switched and the game begins again. Whoever has the most points at the end is the Scarves champion.

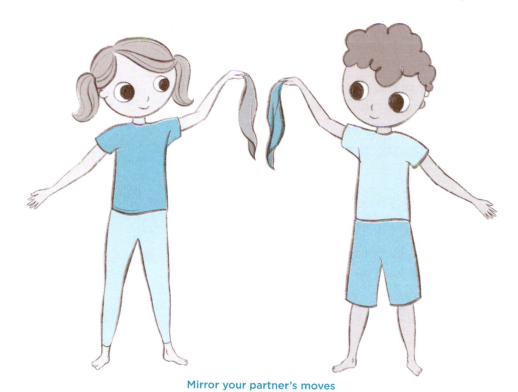

Mirror your partner's moves

PENCILS

What Is Pencils and How Does It help?

Pencils is a fun, focus-based game to play with a friend or partner anytime. Focus-based activities are especially helpful for children who find sitting still to be challenging. Your child will reap the benefits of meditation—as the exercise requires a quiet and focused mind to play—while remaining physically active.

» Also good for: focus

What Do You Need?

- Two new unsharpened pencils (flat on both ends)

TIPS:

- *Play around with different and more challenging ways to suspend the pencil between two partners: fingertips, toes, feet, shoulder-to-shoulder, or back-to-back.*

- *Teachers: This exercise provides a great break during the school day to help refocus a class and build trust and teamwork among peers— with all the advantages of meditation to boot!*

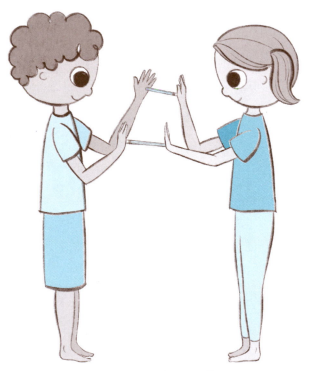

Don't drop the pencils!

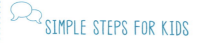

SIMPLE STEPS FOR KIDS

- Begin in a comfortable seated position facing your partner.

- Hold one palm up to face your partner's palm, like a mirror. For example, if Partner One holds up his left palm, Partner Two holds up her right palm.

- Place one pencil between the palms. Gently press palms into the flat ends of the pencil, suspending the pencil in air between the partners' palms.

- Begin to move the pencil around without dropping it.

- Take turns leading.

- Once you feel comfortable moving one pencil, place the second pencil between the other two palms.

- Move each hand in different directions and speeds. Can you move both pencils at once without dropping them?

- Once you feel comfortable moving the two pencils while sitting, stand up and walk around the room, still connected to your partner by the two pencils.

- Can you move around the room and move the pencils in unison without dropping them?

- Have fun with this activity! It is okay if you drop the pencils; it will happen sometimes. Pick them up, refocus, and begin again.

Acknowledgments

First of all, I would like to thank all at Sterling Publishing for believing in this book and getting it out into the world and hands of readers, parents, teachers, and children. I am especially grateful to my editor, Meredith Hale, whose feedback and clever insights shaped my original manuscript into a sparkling gem. This book would not be what it is without you, Meredith, so THANK YOU! And, I'd like to thank the creative team—Lorie Pagnozzi, Shannon Plunkett, Julia Morris, and Elizabeth Lindy— who brought the material to life with skilled design and illustration, as well as production editor Renee Yewdaev and production manager Ellen Day Hudson.

I am indebted to my students who bring me so much joy sharing the magic of yoga, breathing, and meditation with them. My patients and their families approach our sessions with a sense of openness and curiosity during what can typically be a very personal and stressful period. These valuable experiences provide the opportunity to continue growing as a teacher and inspired me to write this book.

Index

About the Author

LISA ROBERTS is a Registered Yoga Teacher and Registered Children's Yoga Teacher, and holds a certificate in Children's Yoga Therapy. She has worked in the pediatric wellness field since 2006 and currently runs the in-patient yoga program at St. Louis Children's Hospital.

Lisa offers professional training, teaching Kids Adaptive and Accessible Yoga to pediatric professionals, parents, and yoga teachers. She is the author of a children's yoga storybook and has developed a line of teaching tools for pediatric yoga teachers, parents, and kids.

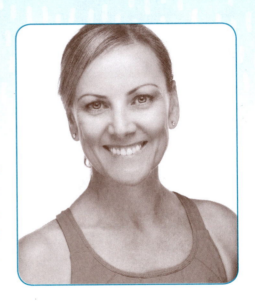

WEBSITE: www.yoyoyogaschool.com
BLOG: http://yoyoyogaschool.com/teaching-tips/blog
FACEBOOK: https://www.facebook.com/yoyoyogaschool
TWITTER: @yoyoyogaschool